"In today's post #MeToo era, so m̲a̲n̲y̲ ̲m̲e̲n̲ ̲a̲r̲e̲ ̲c̲o̲n̲f̲u̲s̲e̲d̲ about what it means to be a man and what women really want. *Conscious Cock* (I especially love this title) is a fantastic primer on what women are asking for. Kristopher has written an easy to follow, real world guide on how to bring consciousness into our sexuality. Women are asking us to get into our heart, without losing a drop of our primal sexuality. This book helps show you the way."

--Jonathan Hudson, Somatic Sexologist
www.SextraordinaryLiving.com

"Kristopher's simple structured approach to relating and sexuality, as well as his clear down-to-earth writing, makes this book a gem for any man wanting to grow the skills and qualities that will garner rave reviews from girlfriends, partners, and wives alike. I recommend this book to all men wishing to become better men, better lovers, and better humans. If any of them does just 10% of what is in *Conscious Cock*, the world will be a better place indeed."

--Philippe Lewis, Sex & Relationship Guide
Exquisite Love Coaching, www.Exquisite.love

"*Conscious Cock* is raw, honest and real. It asks men to step outside of role-playing for the sake of society's expectation of them, and dial into the treasure-trove of pleasure to be had when a guy gets present with his own body and his partner. The "Conscious Cock" is not some disconnected tool to conquer, dominate or service, but rather a sensitive, responsive extension of a whole person. What a radical (and radically important for our times) idea."

--Jennifer Lang M.D., OB/GYN
www.ConsentTheBook.com

"From 15 years as a men's coach I have seen that when men feel wrong about their sexuality they act out their shadow -- either grabbing for power and pleasure or collapsing into despair and isolation. Kristopher's book allows men to bring their sexuality into the light, with simple, actionable tools to reduce shame and create a clear path to deep connection and exciting passion. If this manual existed when I was starting to explore sex, it would have saved me and my male partners a lot of pain!"

--Shana James M.A., Men's Coach
www.ShanaJamesCoaching.com

"Kristopher teaches the kind of sexual intimacy that most women crave from their lovers -- physically, mentally, and emotionally. Through the lens of mindful interactions and compassion, he provides invaluable guidance for men who want to experience conscious intimacy."

-- Jennifer Gunsaullus, PhD, Sociologist & Author of
From Madness to Mindfulness: Reinventing Sex for Women
www.drjennsden.com

"*Conscious Cock* is the book I wish I had as a young man. And it is one that every man should read, no matter what life stage they are in. Kristopher is an engaging and accessible guide through topics of male health, sexuality, and relationships. In the era of #MeToo, Kristopher has brilliantly integrated his embrace of consent culture with a wholehearted affirmation of liberated male sexuality. The book is not only a manual, it is a manifesto for healthy masculinity in a world that needs it now more than ever."

--Dan Mahle, Founder Wholehearted Masculine
www.WholeheartedMasculine.org

"Kristopher really speaks to the heart of what it means to be a man in today's world. He provides practical, insightful, and deeply heartfelt suggestions for how to experience more fulfillment, more understanding, and more intimacy in every aspect of a man's life. *Conscious Cock* will become the textbook to which I refer all of my clients for clear answers that truly every man and his partner are wondering about. I am grateful for Kristopher's brilliant journey into the male experience!"

--Nicole Emma, Intimacy Coach & Sex Educator

"*Conscious Cock* offers an incredibly clear way to address what this culture has needed for a very long time: a guidebook for men that allows them to be 100% who they are without shame or blame, a shift from a sex-negative mindset to a sex-positive one. This book looks at why men struggle with sex, intimacy, and relationships, and presents a new way to move forward. If you are wanting to upgrade your relationship, enhance your sexual performance, increase your capacity to be more authentic and more empowered, and support your partner in doing the same, then this book is for you."

--Laurie Ellington, Open Relationship &
Polyamory Coach, www.poly-coach.com

"Thank you Kris! This book is a must-have for the men who want healthier, happier and hotter relationships AND a huge gift for the women who want their men to show up more fully in partnership. *Conscious Cock* is the ultimate guide to experiencing deeper intimacy."

--Junie Moon, Love Mentor & Author of
Loving the Whole Package, www.CoachJunieMoon.com

"Thank God someone finally wrote such a simple, comprehensive guide to explain the aspects of attraction we never get consciously taught. *Conscious Cock* gives a whole new meaning to the words "fuck my life!" I loved its no holds barred honesty, mixed with understanding that sexual topics, especially ones involving shame, are hard to talk about or even look at. Every time I felt overwhelmed, there was Kristopher, ready with the right words to bring empathy mixed with a heartfelt challenge to 'rise to the occasion' of living my own life."

> --Sara Ness, Founder Authentic Revolution
> www.AuthRev.com

"This book includes all the stuff our parents didn't, and COULDN'T, tell us about! Thanks to Kristopher, it's all in one place, organized, and streamlined for EASY consumption."

> --Mario Singelmann, CEO and Dating Coach,
> Get Game Group Dating Coaching for Men and Women
> www.upyourdatinggame.com

"There comes a time when you are ready to know more and learn more. *Conscious Cock* is just the right book for that. Not only for men but also their girlfriends and partners."

> --Shakun Sethi, Founder, www.Tickle.Life

"*Conscious Cock* is an accessible and relatable sexuality guide for men who love women that is both gentle and understanding as well as fierce and unapologetic. It is a warrior call for men to step up and into what is possible in the realms of intimacy and sex as we co-create the new paradigm of living and loving."

--Juliana Rose Goldstone, Pleasure Activist,
Somatic Sex Educator, Intimacy Coach
www.boldlyembodied.com

CONSCIOUS COCK

The Empowered Sexuality Manual for Men:
Healthy Masculinity, Sex Education &
Communication Tools

KRISTOPHER LOVESTONE

Moons Grove Press
British Columbia, Canada

Conscious Cock:
The Empowered Sexuality Manual for Men:
Healthy Masculinity, Sex Education & Communication Tools

Copyright ©2020 by Kristopher Lovestone
ISBN-13   978-1-77143-407-2
Second Edition

Library and Archives Canada Cataloguing in Publication
Title: Conscious cock : the empowered sexuality manual for men : healthy masculinity,
sex education & communication tools / Kristopher Lovestone.
Names: Lovestone, Kristopher, 1974- author.
Description: Includes bibliographical references.
Identifiers: Canadiana (print) 20190230029 | Canadiana (ebook) 20190230185 |
ISBN 9781771434072 (softcover) | ISBN 9781771434089 (PDF)
Subjects: LCSH: Sex instruction for men. | LCSH: Men—Sexual behavior. |
LCSH: Men—Conduct of life. | LCSH: Masculinity. |
LCSH: Interpersonal communication in men. |
LCSH: Man-woman relationships. | LCGFT: Self-help publications.
Classification: LCC HQ36 .L68 2019 | DDC 613.9/6—dc23

Conscious Cock was first published in February 2019.

Cover artwork credit: cover design & artwork © Kristopher Lovestone
All images contained herein are © Kristopher Lovestone

Disclaimer: SEE YOUR PHYSICIAN. The information in this book is not
intended to replace that of your physician and does not constitute medical advice,
diagnosis or treatment. Do not use this book in place of proper medical care.
Readers are advised to seek professional medical assistance in the event that they
are suffering from any medical problem and before starting any exercise program.
All health questions concerning yourself or anyone else, must initially be
addressed by your doctor, physician or other qualified health professional.

Extreme care has been taken by the author to ensure that all information
presented in this book is accurate and up to date at the time of publishing.
Neither the author nor the publisher can be held responsible for any errors or
omissions. Additionally, neither is any liability assumed for damages resulting
from the use of the information contained herein.

All rights reserved. No part of this publication may be reproduced, stored in a
retrieval system or transmitted in any form or by any means, electronic,
mechanical, photocopying, recording or otherwise without the express written
permission of the author/publisher, except in the case of brief and accurately
credited quotations embodied in critical articles or reviews.

www.ConsciousCock.com

Moons Grove Press is an imprint
of CCB Publishing: www.ccbpublishing.com

Moons Grove Press
British Columbia, Canada
www.moonsgrovepress.com

This book is dedicated to

The balancing of the masculine and feminine,

To the empowerment of all people,

To the end of oppression and sexual shame,

And to the rise of an era when sex is seen

As a beautiful and healthy thing.

Conscious Cock Is Medicine

A POEM BY ALANA LOUISE MAY[1]
http://lanalouisemay.com

If men understood the value of a well fucked woman they would have no choice but to prioritize their sexual evolution. If you understood that having a well fucked woman on your side was the formula to succeeding in life, in every realm and every kingdom it would become your religion, religiously giving her everything you've got, on your knees thrusting in prayer, hymns flowing from her hips to her lips a gospel choir conducted by your conductor, symphonies as sweet as an angel's breath written by your caress.

Taking her deeper than the material, the mundane, the physical, undressing her body, mind and soul, she is your ticket to success. The most valuable asset you could ever invest in, your embodied evolution, your sexual consciousness. She will ooze all over your existence, lusciously dripping warm and melting, lubricating your life, the ease within your flow, the Lakshmi to your abundance, the magic behind your power.

A moisturized life, gleaming in the glory of her erotically charged radiance. The remedy to your everything, a slathered on savior, the coconut oil of the human variety.

Apply liberally.

Her creative energy that you have assisted in its activation, stirred up within her cauldron, will birth your every dream

---

[1] Conscious Cock Is Medicine by Alana Louise May is reproduced with permission.

into reality. Your conscious cock is like a wizard's wand, interacting with her magic to manifest. Co-creating a new world with every breath, pulse and moan.

You have the power to be the god she calls her own. Taking her to heights most holy upon sweaty sheets. You can be the moon to her tides, eclipsing her preoccupation with the mind, you can blow the wind into her sails and lift her up high to explore the oceans of the skies, the power in your body vibrating, attuned, refined. Divorcing her from unconsciousness and reuniting her with the divine, helping her become clarified.

Taking her into timeless trance states where her body lay beneath your own, yet her psyche is in another dimensional time zone, reciting poetry straight from God's kiss, a lyrical psychic physicist, delivering wisdom straight from creation's mind back in her body for dinner time.

You can be a part of miracles like that on the daily if you desire. When you heal one of us you heal us all. Conscious cock is medicine and we are all suffering from our unfilled prescriptions.

We have become diseased from a lack of connection, from ourselves, from each other, from the earth, from the feminine. Now is the time for our reclamation. If you are into transformation and ignoring your sexuality you are sorely mistaken, our evolution relies on our full bodied and souled integration.

You can't possibly know the power you're denying. All the women you're depriving. Conscious Cock is Medicine.

Contents

Preface

Many ancient cultures had a concept of reverence for the male and female genitalia and their power to give life, pleasure and union with the Divine. Sexuality was celebrated as an integral part in our existence and a way to connect with the Sacred.

In the English language our sexual shame is so embedded that we do not have any terms of reverence for the male or female genitalia. We have only either derogatory terms (dick, cock) or medical terms (penis, phallus)! There are no words of appreciation, respect or admiration, no words of beauty, adoration or veneration. The penis is most commonly cited to infer indignation and strong disapproval.

Our language determines our ability to conceptualize and see. With a lack of words of regard for the penis, we remain trapped in our vision of it as a negative thing. Recently some infiltration of a positive word for the penis from Sanskrit has begun. The word "lingam" is usually heard in relation to Tantric lingam massage. Roughly translated as "shaft of light," it refers to the male God Shiva and more specifically to his penis as the source of all life and creation. Relatedly the Sanskrit word "yoni" has come into slightly common usage in English as a word of appreciation and respect for the female genitalia, meaning "divine passage," "place of origin" or "temple."

These are powerful thought stimulators to help us move away from a sex-negative culture to a sex-positive one where we can put down the shackles of sexual shame given to us by our caregivers, role models, churches, communities and popular media.

Today many people are leaning into an inner feeling that *sex is sacred*, but without words to refer to even our sexual organs in a sacred manner, it is a steep hill to climb.

As such, I offer you *Conscious Cock*. It is a reclaiming of a derogatory term to make it positive. It is a normalizing of something previously considered an insult or curse word. It is an opening to allow us to consider the amazing beautiful power that is possible in a healthy, balanced view of masculinity, and it is ultimately the source of life from which we all come and without which our race could not exist.

In the wake of #MeToo and the great public uncovering of the scope of oppression, abuse, harassment and shaming of women, it is of the utmost importance that we develop ways to foster positive, healthy masculinity, and we must start with our language… for only with a word can complete thoughts coalesce.

I encourage you not to use words that refer to the genitals as derogatory words. Don't call someone a "dick" or a "pussy" or an "asshole" to slander them. These words refer to our genitals and we should reframe our concept of the value of our genitals to make them precious rather than derogatory. Only then can we begin to cast off our shame surrounding our sexuality.

Introduction

This book is for heterosexual men who want to craft the relationship of their dreams--whether they are currently single or already in a relationship. They're good guys who are an asset to the world. They are doing everything they can do to be the best they can be. They want to have a better relationship and get more of what they really want out of it, and they don't want to be a jerk.

They know how pervasive abuse and harassment of women is, and they don't want to be a part of that system. They want to be a part of the solution but simultaneously want to get more of their deep inner needs met rather than acting some part or playing some role.

They have some hidden dissatisfaction with their relationship. They want it to be better, hotter and more able to support them to unfold and evolve into who they want to become in the future. However, they don't know anyone who is truly successful in relationships to look up to and learn from. They feel like they are in a void--trying to go it alone without solidarity from other rising men to lean on.

I know. I've been there, and I want to invite you to be a part of the change.

I grew up an only child to a single mom who was in one failed relationship after another for my entire life. I literally lived through six divorces in my childhood, and in them I got to witness all the bullshit, all the failed connections, all the pain and all the dysfunctional patterns that people live with. I saw firsthand how brutal and manipulative people can be to each other, and I decided that I wasn't going to end up like that. I wished I'd had a manual to follow to succeed in my relationships and sex life, but I only had role models of men who I didn't want to be like to offer me reference points on my journey.

At 10 years old I started educating myself about relationships, sex and communication. As a young adult I had my fair share of failed relationships, and even ended up feeling suicidal when I realized I wasn't getting what I really wanted and felt I was at a dead end. With dedication to learning and expanding my repertoire of tools through over 30 years of study and practice, I eventually broke through to a whole new and easy way of relating that yields amazing satisfaction and sexual pleasure.

If I can do it, anyone can do it, but it's easier if you have someone show you the way so you don't have to recreate the wheel. I started out so shy, repressed, ashamed and scared that I couldn't even talk to women. All my initial forays into sex and relationships were a failure. But, by learning the techniques that I'm going to share with you in this book, I've been able to build the relationship and sex life of my dreams. I now live with my wife (who is my best friend and partner) of almost 15 years in the most inspiring relationship of anyone I know--with complete acceptance, openness and unconditional support of the true unabridged reality of each other. It's sexier now than it has ever been, and it keeps getting hotter and more adventurous because of the tools I present here.

Now I help men and their partners to construct the

relationship that they really want. I've distilled these 30+ years of relationship and sex study into a simple, radical system that helps men to get past roadblocks that they don't often even know they have without need for therapy or psychoanalysis. By shining the light on blind spots and employing simple to learn real-world tools, I help them to break out of toxic and repetitive patterns to uncover and begin achieving what they really want in their relationships.

Usually when you boil it all down it ultimately has to do with sex and intimacy. His deepest desires and needs go unmet and he ends up feeling like he's living someone else's life. That leads to resentment, frustration, complacency, depression or addiction; and the relationship suffers in a downward spiral of a negative reinforcing feedback loop.

When we uncover the truth about what he wants and then give him tools to help make that happen, we reverse the direction. Then in an upward spiral of a positive reinforcing feedback loop the sky becomes the limit. All topics are on the table and anything is possible. For many it's the first hope and inspiration they've felt since the honeymoon phase of the relationship wore off.

Conscious Cock is about embodying our masculinity in a mindful way. It is a radical response to traditional toxic masculinity. It is about embracing our sexuality consciously rather than repressing it or using it to abuse or oppress women. It is about bringing out our full potential to be kickass human beings who support and empower our loved ones and know how to be mature and take care of our own needs and desires. It is about empowering men to become the best versions of themselves rather than the unfulfilled, apathetic, addicted, oppressive or desperate men all around us.

It's about radically breaking free from the norm and building a new (and sexy!) masculinity based on deep authenticity, transparency and integrity. When you know how to truly be real while simultaneously not being domineering or pathetic, the door to unlimited possibilities opens before you.

What do you want? How would you design the relationship structure of your dreams? What type of intimacy do you most desire with your partner? Do you feel unfulfilled? Do you feel like you never really sync with your partner? Are you afraid to share your fantasies, your desires or your true feelings? Do you feel castrated or paralyzed because you don't know how to proceed, and you don't want to do anything wrong?

These are the common things I hear from all the men I work with, and lucky for you that you have this book in your hands because it offers you a road map to get from where you are now to the road to your unique idea of relationship success and sexual fulfillment.

You don't have to be a robot. You don't have to do what everyone else is doing, and *you don't have to do it alone*!

Conscious Cock is also about building community between rising men. Through our online discussion group and weekly group calls (See Appendix B at the back of this book), we offer each other a priceless jewel: a safe place to talk about what is really going on for us without fear of backlash. We offer each other support, encouragement and solidarity as we learn from each other on our parallel paths to relationship and sex life success. Being engaged with a group of men who've got your back is powerful, and it makes you more powerful, confident and less needy of female approval.

Usually men never talk about their sex lives or relationships unless it is in a joking or derogatory manner or in a session with a therapist. *Conscious Cock* changes that. We make this conversation normal rather than weird, and we give the tools (and the support to learn to master them) that work in this modern day and age. When we embody this type of healthy masculinity, we answer the calling that the world has today for men to act consciously.

Relationships are messy, and there are no guarantees, but when men gather to support each other in positive ways that foster growth rather than enforce conformity, amazing things happen. Lives change and the future changes with it. What could be better than a bright relationship future where your true inner sexual desires are embraced and supported by your partner and you don't feel like you are playing some role that you don't want to play! The *Conscious Cock* way to get there is by facilitating both you and your partner to get real with each other, destroy the common relationship and communication challenges, and give you solid actionable sex education and exercises to empower your love life.

Welcome to the Conscious Cock Brotherhood.

How This Book Is Organized

This book is intended to be read from start to finish. Of course, you can jump around and look at the material you want to look at, but the tools and materials are presented in a sequence that allows you to build upon what you've learned in the previous chapter. I highly recommend that you make a personal commitment to yourself to do what it takes to start at the beginning and proceed sequentially all the way through to the end of the book.

It's perfectly fine to put the book down for a while to integrate what you've read and then come back and continue with the next chapter when you are ready. Rushing and pushing yourself will only reduce your success rate.

The book is divided into five main sections:

1) Installing Some Upgrades
2) Understanding Your Partner
3) Increasing Your Sex Education
4) Stoking the Fire in Your Relationship
5) Improving Your Sex Technique

Each section builds on the materials presented in the previous sections so that by the time you finally get to the sex tools you will have a firm foundation in self-awareness, authenticity and communication to be able to handle the sex tools in a truly conscious masculine manner.

At the end of the book are the appendices. These

include worksheets, exercises and links to help you "get" the material and apply it to your own life and circumstances. If you just read the book, you will theoretically understand the concepts, but if you also do the work then you will understand the concepts through practice. To be a Conscious Cock, you need to be able to walk the talk, not just talk it. The world doesn't need yet another man spewing forth opinions that he hasn't put into practice in his own life and succeeded at, so I encourage you to do each worksheet or exercise when they are cited in the book.

Note: You can copy the worksheets on a photocopier so that you can have many blank worksheets to work from. This enables you to do the exercises multiple times, to share them with friends and to have your partner do them too. Of course, you can also just use a pen or pencil and fill them out right in the book to keep everything handy in one place.

I encourage you to keep a pen with this book and underline things that you like. Fold over the corners of pages that you liked or impacted you and write notes and thoughts in the margins. Use this as a workbook to sort out your thoughts and feel what comes up for you, and if you want more support then join the brotherhood by joining our Facebook group and online community where I host group calls and coaching sessions each week. If you want to ask me a question directly, I am available for one-on-one coaching sessions. More information is available on my website at www.consciouscock.com.

Section 1:

Install Some Upgrades

Chapter 1: Mindset

Let's get started with the first tool: setting your mindset for success.

For any of this to work at all, you must open your mind to the chance that doing something different might work. Part of that means making yourself acknowledge that you don't have it all figured out, that you've made mistakes, and you are willing and want to do things differently and better now. Not some hypothetical thing, but a reality.

I invite you to commit to the fulfillment of an empowered and deliciously sexy life. Decide here and now, that you are going to open your mind and try these tools. Let them work their magic, even if they sound weird or impossible for you. Let go of your judgments. Set your mind state for success and notice and prevent yourself from self-sabotage. Commit to the process! Try on these tools and you'll find that they work wonders. Commit to following through and putting into action what I will share here with you--for your happiness and for the good of your sex life and relationships, and everyone touched by them. And then, set this goal for yourself. Decide here and now that you are going to fuck your life.

When I say I want you to "fuck your life," I mean I want you to be bold in your life. Don't just let life happen to you--silently taking whatever comes. Be assertive. Be bold. Be ballsy. Take some control and make some joy happen in your life. Enjoy being alive by claiming your power and having sex with life. I want you to take pleasure in getting out of life the juicy joy that you want to get out of it. You deserve it. No one is responsible for your happiness except you. If you aren't happy with your life, you can change it. Start by giving yourself permission to take chances, be bold, and speak your mind. Be like the cocky rooster going around strutting his stuff. Don't shrink from life. Rise to it. Meet it.

You could be dead! But you're not. You're here now because you want something better, so commit to action, give it your root power and make it into reality. Your sexual energy is the fire of your life and your ability to give life. Use it to empower your life. Let your sexual energy fill you with courage and with strength. Then use it to extract exquisite pleasure from doing the things in your life that you want and taking pleasure from being an adult with the freedom to make up his own mind and do what he wants to do.

This doesn't mean be a jerk. But it does mean claiming your sexual power. Don't just sit by and let life happen to you. Don't just lay on your back and take it. Fuck your life. Take charge and move some pieces around the board so that you get more satisfaction from every day. Enjoy your life, just like you enjoy getting pleasure from sex. How are you going to get what you want from your life today? Make more money? Do a thing you love to do but never get around to? Make love to your partner? Achieve a goal from your bucket list that you keep putting off? Go out and fuck your life. Make it scream and love every creamy juicy delicious moment of it. Commit to the process and then stand up in your own life and have sex with it.

I run a private discussion group on Facebook called the Conscious Cock Brotherhood where rising men can congregate to share what they are going through and offer and get support that they are lacking in their normal worldly life. At this point I'd like to invite you to go join the group and introduce yourself there, share where you are from and what you are going through and what you want to achieve by reading this book.

I encourage you to be raw and completely honest and share what's really going on for you. I moderate the group and ensure that it is a safe-space for us to be real and authentic with each other.

Then think about what you really enjoy and want in life and then go out today and take your life and fuck it. Do something healthy and satisfying that you really want to do for yourself and derive joy from it. Do it for your own joy and satisfaction at being a man and being alive. Take it. It's your life. If you don't do it, no one is going to do it for you.

Chapter 2: Natural Male Enhancement

A lot of men joke about Viagra, but it's a serious subject. A lot of men, including me, are insecure about the size of their cock, the hardness of their erections, the length of their stamina during intercourse or the power or amount of their ejaculations. Especially if you watch porn and see all these men with unrealistic monster cocks and mistakenly believe even subconsciously that they are anything like normal. They aren't. Most of them are taking Viagra to be able to maintain their erections that long and have spent years increasing their penis size.

Feeling insecure about our size and performance ability is not a joke. A lot of us carry these issues around like weights on our shoulders--worrying or sad that we aren't as good as we want to be. A lot of us are afraid to be seen naked and like to cover ourselves from our lovers because we aren't happy with what we've got.

Let me speak to that part of you that has ever felt inadequate or wished you were different than you are. I know men never talk about this stuff, and it might be uncomfortable to even read anything about it, but I assure you if you just take this information in with the mindset that you might find some valuable information here to help you then you'll feel better because of it.

Let's get right to it. I'm going to tell you a fact. You can change your cock and your sexual performance. You can. You may not know it, but by doing specific exercises you can literally increase the hardness of your erections, increase your stamina during intercourse, prevent premature ejaculation, and increase the power and amount of your ejaculations. It's true. You don't need Viagra. You don't need the latest plastic surgery fad of a cock transplant. You just need to know what the exercises are and then do them regularly. It's not rocket science. It's a form of working out your cock and the muscles that drive it.

The exercises that I share here will give you increased erection and ejaculation strength, help you to get an erection when you want, make yourself hard and help you stay hard and will help you reach orgasm during the times when it's hard to reach. If you ever dribble a drop or two of urine after peeing, then you *need* to do these exercises already for your own health.

Did you know that the single biggest reason people end up in nursing homes when they get old is because they can't hold their bladder? They can't keep themselves from peeing, so they end up wetting their bed and peeing themselves and must be put into diapers and then an assisted living facility. It's heartbreaking and completely avoidable. You can add another ten to twenty years of independent free living to your life by simply doing these exercises!

Aside from that however, probably the biggest benefit of doing these exercises is that you will last longer during sex and be better able to reach orgasm when you want it-- because sometimes it can be hard to get there. You'll also be better able to hold off orgasm until you choose to release. Another awesome benefit is that they can enable you to have multiple orgasms during the same single lovemaking session. You can learn to keep your cock hard after having your first orgasm and keep going until you recover your energy and then can have a second orgasm. Let me tell you from personal experience that it's delightful for your partner and she'll thank you for it.

The basic exercise is called PC muscle exercises, pelvic floor exercises, or Kegels, and you can do them anywhere and any time since you don't need any actual weights. There are many variations of a Kegel exercise routine. I recommend you commit to doing the exercise every time that you take a shower alone or go to the bathroom. Just use the toilet rather than the urinal so that you can relax in privacy, and you aren't taking time out of your day.

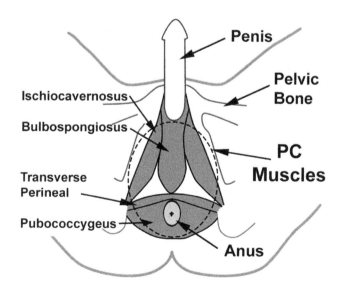

1. Locate your PC muscles.

The PC muscles are actually a group of four distinct muscles that surround the base of the cock inside the body. In the diagram above you can see that the ischiocavernosus, bulbospongiosus, transverse perineal and pubococcygeus muscles (whew, that's a mouthful!) are all together referred to as the "PC muscles". They work together to support erections, stop the flow of urine and squeeze your anus shut all at the same time. Simply squeezing to stop the flow of urine while peeing is contracting these four muscles together.

Note in the following image that the PC muscles are suspended like a net from the pubic bone to the tail bone, holding our organs up and tightly inside the body. The urethra and the anus pass through the PC muscles.

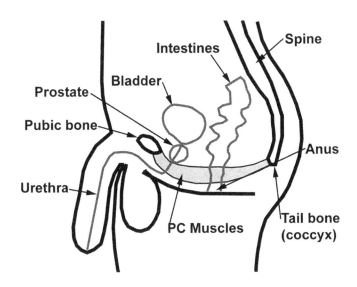

Squeeze your PC muscles by stopping peeing the next time you go to the bathroom. Note the sensations inside your pelvis when you stop the urine midstream. They will help you to recognize the PC muscles. You can press a couple fingers up behind your balls while you practice squeezing the PC muscles a few times, and you should feel the muscles tighten with your fingertips.

While you squeeze your PC muscles notice if you are also contracting your belly, abs, thighs or butt. If you are then try relaxing them and only contract the PC muscles. You need to be able to differentiate between the PC muscles and the muscles of the belly, abs, thighs and butt so that you can contract only the PC muscles.

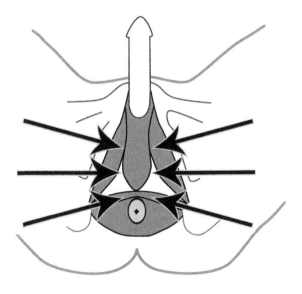

2. How much to flex the PC muscles

To do the exercise properly you must learn to flex the PC muscles the correct amount. Flexing too much can easily injure your PC muscles, and flexing them too little won't actually exercise the muscles enough to have a positive effect. I can't stress this enough: you do not want to injure your PC muscles by overworking them! Flexing them too hard too many times will hurt them, and you will be injured.

Let go of our common tendency to go at challenges aggressively here! Gentle repetition is better than trying too hard and hurting yourself!

To begin exercising your PC muscles, aim to find a gentle to mid-strength contraction of between 30 to 50% flex. For reference, a 100% flex contraction would be squeezing as hard as you can possibly squeeze, while a 0% contraction would be not squeezing at all.

One way to find this ideal beginning contraction intensity is to experiment while urinating. The 30% point is just about enough contraction to stop the flow of urine *and no more!* When beginning your PC muscles workout routine, aim for gentle to mid-strength contractions in this 30% to 50% contraction intensity zone.

3. Beginning exercise routine

A good beginning PC muscles exercise routine is to do five to ten of the 30% to 50% contraction intensity squeezes for five seconds each followed by five to ten seconds of relaxing and breathing, repeated three to five times per week. Another way to say that is five to ten repetitions (also known as "reps") for five seconds, three to five days a week.

It's very important to relax and breathe deeply in between each contraction, and you *must* remember to aim for 30% to 50% intensity contractions rather than squeezing too hard!

Remember it's best to consult a medical professional before beginning any exercise routine, and it's also better to be do less intensity workouts reliably than it is to do harder intensity workouts irregularly and infrequently.

4. Increasing the intensity of the workout

As the PC muscles strengthen with the beginner routine, the workout intensity can be increased gradually. A goal is to do 50 reps of five second contractions over the course of six weeks and then take a week off before continuing at 50 reps per workout.

For example, the intensity can be increased like this:

Week 1: 5 reps per workout
Week 2: 10 reps per workout
Week 3: 20 reps per workout
Week 4: 30 reps per workout
Week 5: 40 reps per workout
Week 6: 50 reps per workout
Week 7: Total break

If at any time you experience a feeling of having worked out too hard, take a break for a week and then go back to the number of reps from the previous week. For example, if you were doing 30 reps per workout and felt like it was too much, then take a week off and then return to working out the following week at 20 reps per workout.

This is general information and is not intended to be a customized workout routine nor medical advice. To ensure that you don't hurt yourself always err on the side of caution and conservative workouts, and consult a medical professional.

5. Intermediate level workouts

If you reach 50 reps per workout and feel like it's no longer challenging, you can go in multiple directions. From here it's best to customize your workout routine with the help of a trained coach, but generally speaking you can increase the length of contractions, increase the number of reps, and increase the number of workouts you do per day/week.

For example, you can work up to holding the contractions for longer periods of time, as in *working up to*:

50 reps of 10 second contractions

5 reps of 50 second contractions

1 rep of a 100 second contraction

To increase the number of reps, you could for example *work up to* 100 reps of 5 second contractions. Or even more!

To increase the number of workouts, you could increase from one set per day, three to five times per week to two sets per day three to five times per week, or even work up to three sets per day three to five times per week.

The key is always to go slow, be conservative, and take a week off every six weeks or any time you are feeling over-worked.

Another intermediate level option is to learn to distinguish between the anterior and posterior portions of your PC muscles--meaning the parts that are more in front or more in back. It is possible to squeeze the group of muscle fibers that close off the urethra and relax the group of muscle fibers that open up the anus and vice versa.

In other words you can gain control and specificity of the muscle fiber groups that control the penile contractions separately from the muscle fiber groups that control anal contractions. An exercise for this is to go to the bathroom when you need to both urinate and defecate at the same time. Then while on the toilet practice doing one but not the other for a moment and then switching. For example, try to hold your ass tightly closed while you let yourself urinate. Then switch and try to hold your urine while letting your ass relax and poop.

It may sound strange, but learning to differentiate between the penis and anus PC muscles and control them separately is an excellent intermediate exercise to help give you mastery and powerful control over your orgasms!

There are many more PC muscle workout types, so if you get this far and are excited to continue, please get a good coach. If you don't know where to start, you can contact me. The benefits of keeping this musculature toned are numerous. You'll likely experience much greater erectile strength, ability to last longer in bed, ability to get an erection when you want one, and ability to hold off your orgasm until you *decide* that you want to release!

If you want to make a big improvement in your sex life and to put some energy into taking care of your own health, then commit to your transformation and happiness and do these exercises every day for the next 30 days. I challenge you to do it. It doesn't take any time out of your day, and it will significantly improve your experience of sex and your sexual power.

If you want to go even farther and increase the length and girth of your penis at the same time that you increase the strength of your erections and ability to last longer in bed, then you need to do jelqing in addition to Kegels. Jelqing is a manual exercise, similar to masturbation, where you *carefully* work-out the tissues of the penis. Much like weight-training in a gym, through repeated exercise the tissues increase in size. Men can literally gain length and girth to both their flaccid and erect penis states in months of careful exercise. This is an advanced technique that is beyond the scope of this book, but for more information see "Recommended Resources" in Appendix A. You must have professional supervision however because if you do the exercises wrong you can hurt your cock, and I guarantee you don't want a cock injury that you'll have to recover from!

Remember to fuck your life and start and keep doing the Kegel exercises every day for the next 30 days to boost your sexual confidence and performance ability significantly. If you have any questions, please visit and join the Conscious Cock Brotherhood Facebook group and post them there. See Appendix A.

Chapter 3: Wield the Power of Consent

This chapter is all about how to wield the power of consent to empower your relationships and sex life. Lots of men roll their eyes when someone mentions consent and boundaries, but I think that's only because they don't really understand it. Perhaps they think they understand it but are letting their preconceived notions tell them what to think, rather than learning about it with an open mind and then having an informed opinion. Thinking that you know everything when you haven't spent the time to learn about it is just the kind of thing that unconscious jerks do. I encourage you to take the conscious cock path and open your mind and take this information about how wielding the power of consent can empower your sex life!

Let's approach it this way. Do you ever try to take care of other people's feelings? Do you ever go along with things because that's what you feel is expected of you? Do you ever say yes when really you want to say no? Is it hard for you to say no? Is it hard for you to hear a "no" when you make a request to a woman? Do you take it personally? Do you pressure her to change her mind?

All these things are symptoms of not understanding how to wield the power of consent. When you truly understand what it means and how to employ it in your own life, then your entire outlook shifts. This is one of the most powerful self-empowerment lessons that we will be covering in this book. It affects every area of one's life and can completely revolutionize your outlook on the future and your ability to get what you want. It's about finding your true inner voice, being able to communicate it clearly, being able to solicit other people's true inner voices, and being able to take their no's as gracefully as their yes's.

Most of us nice men never set boundaries. We just go with the flow and try to make everyone like us. Seldom do we draw a line and say, "This is where I stand, this is what I'm OK with and what I'm not OK with. If you want to be with me, then I need you to respect this line." I like to think of a boundary like a fence around a playground. Within the fence it's OK to play. It's alright to play right up to the fence and even lean into it and bounce off it. When you know what area is OK to play in, you can relax when you are in that area. It takes away nervousness and doubt because you have a clear line. In this sense a boundary is a thing of liberation because it sets you free to fully inhabit playing within the playground.

Imagine that we are talking about sex with a woman. Let's say hypothetically that this woman is more sexually adventurous or experienced than you. You are never sure what she's going to do, and you are sometimes afraid she's going to do something you don't like. So, you check in with yourself and determine that you don't want to do anything that causes you pain or limits your motion, so you set a boundary that says that it's not OK to hurt you or tie you up in any way. That boundary, assuming she respects it, allows you both to relax into playing anywhere in the playground that it defines: sex and sensuality that feels good and is free of bondage.

If she respects your boundary then she builds trust

with you. Of course, your boundary can be different in the real world. This is just a hypothetical example. Maybe you don't ever want to have anal sex or to be dominated or to go down on her. Whatever it is, it's OK to have your preferences, and I encourage you to set boundaries *so that they exist,* and your partner can get to know what you like and don't like and can know where it's safe to play with you.

By contrast, not knowing where the boundary is causes doubt and insecurity. If you aren't sure what's OK, then you can end up being nervous or too cautious or worse… accidentally doing something that she really doesn't want you to do. It's better to be clear and make agreements by setting and honoring boundaries than randomly shooting in the dark and hoping it works out well.

To wield the power of consent, you need to set boundaries and have your partner set boundaries with you *and then honor them.* Then as you play in your agreed upon playground, you get to see if your partner is meeting your needs and building trust with you and she gets to see if you honor her preferences, which builds trust with her. As trust builds you may feel comfortable moving the fence to allow a bigger playground with more options for play. In other words, if you have built sufficient trust you may feel comfortable exploring your "maybes" with each other. In this manner boundaries are also dynamic and evolving, meaning that you can move them if someone meets or exceeds your expectations.

All this depends on being able to say "yes" and state the things that you want to do, and to be able to say "no" to the things that you don't want to do. If someone can't say "no" then the reality is that their "yes" is meaningless and impotent. If they can't say "no" then it's difficult to trust their "yes." But if you can clearly say "no" you give people the gift of understanding how to work with you. Each "no" is useful information that helps them to navigate their relationship with you. It's like a dance, and as you get the hang of saying "no," your "yes" becomes more powerful because it means something. It works both ways, for both you and her.

It entails both learning to have a powerful "yes" and "no" yourself and learning how to receive a "no" from her. Learning how to honor her "no" by thanking her for taking care of herself and being honest with you.

We men have a tough situation in our culture. We are expected to be the initiators—the ones who approach and invite sexual experiences--yet we are not taught how to handle receiving a "no!" Because of that it feels scary and risky to approach and invite because she may not welcome or reciprocate our advances and we may end up feeling fundamentally rejected. Learning not to take the "no" personally nor take it as "rejection," but rather use the "no" as a navigational aid is a skill that is learned through practice!

It helps to lighten up, not take ourselves too seriously and have a playful mannerism. Also redefining success is key. If you define success as her saying "yes" to your invitation, then of course you'll feel rejected if she says "no." However defining success simply as having the guts to *make the invitation*…regardless of her reaction to it…is much more empowering. Simply putting yourself out there and taking a chance means that you are being brave and taking a risk to maybe get something you want. That is true success because you are demonstrating that your desires are worth going after! Not trying is the only failure.

There's so much more to this than we can cover in this short chapter, so I am going to invite you to dive deeper into this by listening to the audio recording of my "Boundaries & Consent: 6 rules to empower your life" workshop. See the recommended resources link in Appendix A in the back of this book.

I strongly encourage you to set aside an hour to listen to the workshop before you proceed to the next chapter. It will give you life-changing tools that will empower you to alter the course of your future by getting *more of what you really want* while simultaneously doing less of what you don't want to do. I highly recommend that you listen to it with your partner or share it with her after so that you both get the vocabulary into your language and can use it to improve your relationship with each other. But be aware, many people have huge AHA moments that change their lives forever... liberating them from chains they didn't know they were carrying! It's a strong pillar upon which we will base much of the learning in this book, and you can listen to it in your car or on your phone. Then please share any questions, comments, successes and failures in the Facebook group (link in Appendix A), and make sure to keep going with your Kegels and remembering to fuck your life every single day!

Chapter 4: Saying the Unsaid

Up until now we've talked about setting your mindset, improving your erection control and strength, and understanding consent and boundaries through a self-empowerment perspective. The next thing we need to cover is more fundamental to our ability to be real with our partner so that we can have a hope to get what we really want in our relationship.

Can you remember any time when you knew (your internal voice of guidance) that you should say something to your partner? Whether it was something you felt you needed to get off your chest, something that you did that you wanted to apologize for, something you thought but never had the courage to share, or some fantasy that you would like to have with her one day.

The art of "saying the unsaid," sharing something you've been "withholding," or revealing your inner world is quite possibly the single most important thing that you can ever learn to do. This is relationship alchemy here! If you have ever left something unsaid and kept it to yourself when you felt like you should have told your partner, then this is something you'll be able to understand.

There are two pitfalls: saying too much and saying too little. The ideal is to be tactful and not bludgeon your partner with inconsideration, and at the same time not say so little as to lie by omission. I'm going to show you how you can bring up any of the things that you have ever left unsaid so that they stop nagging you and so that you can build trust and faith with your partner.

I'm sure that you can imagine a scenario that could involve not admitting something to your partner that you really feel like you should tell her... and then if she finds out by accident somehow, then suddenly you look like a liar because you never shared it. For example, let's say you ran into an ex-girlfriend who your partner doesn't like, and you sat down for a minute and chatted, but you never told your partner. If she somehow finds out--say from a friend who saw you that day and mentions it to her--you are going to look like an untrustworthy liar in her eyes! These types of situations can be avoided by learning how to say the things that you are leaving unsaid in a prompt and tactful way.

Now let me give you another bad way the above example could play out. This time let's say she didn't find out on her own. Let's say that it just nags you and you keep thinking about it, and you really want to clear the air and get it off your chest so that you can relax with her in an atmosphere of full disclosure. It builds up to a breaking point inside you and suddenly one day you just blurt out, "I had coffee with my ex last week."

Just shocking her like that can prevent her from having a positive response or from responding in the way that you would like her to respond because the shock can trigger her fight or flight reaction. You probably want her to appreciate you for being honest with her, but instead she might react negatively from the shock of you just blurting it out at her suddenly with no warning or context.

The solution to both examples is to become a master in the art of saying the unsaid.

It's not hard. You just need to learn these three steps.

- First, set the context and get her attention. Tell her that there is something that you haven't told her but that you want to tell her, and that the reason you haven't told her is that you are afraid that she will... (and then tell her what you are afraid of, like for example, you fear that she'll get mad at you and break up with you).

- Second, tell her what you want to have happen by telling her, for example: "What I hope is that by telling you this, you'll see that I respect you and want to be honest with you and have no secrets between us, so that we can build a relationship on a foundation of trust--even if it's hard sometimes."

- Third, tell her the thing that you haven't said, and let the cards fall where they may. This is where most people lock up in fear or go on forever and ever, but if you want to have a real relationship of deep connection you must be able to handle the turbulent waters to get to the bliss of smooth sailing. Just make it short and succinct. Just one or two sentences is enough. Anything more has too much "story" in it.

The idea here is to give her context before you say the thing, which helps to put her in a state of openness and maybe even empathy for you. Prepare her and give her a handle to hold on to and communicate to her what you'd like to have happen by making yourself vulnerable and saying the unsaid thing to her.

Let's summarize it for clarity

1. There's something that I want to tell you that I haven't because I'm afraid that you are going to react by (…)

2. What I would like to have happen by telling you this is that you or we (…)

3. The thing that I haven't told you is (…)

It's simple, and once you get it, you'll never forget it and you'll be able to use it in all aspects of your life to clear the air and communicate those difficult things and hard truths that you really feel you need to say. It's an empowering tool to build character and give you a chance to build a strong foundation of trust and honesty in your relationships. It helps you to foster an atmosphere in which sacred juicy sexuality can take root, but more on that in the coming chapters! In the meantime, if you want more help working out how to bring up something that's particularly hard for you to bring up, please go to Appendix B at the back of this book to find a worksheet that you can do as many times as you need to prepare yourself to bring it up and clear the air, and see Chapter 25 where we adapt the technique to bring up sexual activities that you would like to do with your partner.

Chapter 5: Style Update

Your personal style and appearance matters. There's no way around it. If you want to have more and better sex with your partner, then you must be able to take an honest look at yourself and see yourself from an outsider's perspective with a new set of eyes.

One of the awesome things about women is that it usually matters more to them how you take care of yourself, than how much you weigh or how handsome you are or how flat your stomach is. If you make yourself look nice, they often don't care about extra pounds, wrinkles or years. If she loves you it's not because you look like a Greek God. She responds to multiple facets about you, foremost of which is how you treat her and how you make her feel, not your body shape. That's good news for us!

Notice I said, "How you make her feel." This includes her noticing how you look, how you smell, how you taste, how you sound, and how your hands feel when you touch her. All her senses are important!

How long has it been since you refreshed your style? Do you have a style? Or have you been so beaten down or busy in your life that your haircut and appearance and teeth are the last things on your mind? Even though most men put it last on their list, it's one of the most obvious things about you to your partner and everyone else who sees you. How old is your underwear? How old are your shirts? Your shoes? If they are worn, stained, tattered or ripped then think about how that comes across to other people and how they perceive you. Since you are making a change in your life by reading this book, give yourself permission to update your look, your wardrobe and your hairstyle!

Google a hair salon in your area – not grandpa's barber – and go to it and notice the women stylists there and make an appointment with the one who you like the best. Do this even if you are resistant to the idea! It may take courage. Go do it because it may be outside of your comfort zone, but it's worth it for the confidence boost it will give you and how it will likely improve how your partner responds to you. Find a female stylist who you like and then go and tell her that you need her help and want a refresh… an update… and to make you look handsome! If you have a beard, consider changing the style a bit and making it look more intentional and well kept. Let the stylist help you and then tip her well. Enjoy her attention and her touch as a bonus.

Then go to a men's fashion store that's a little more upscale than your current style. Find a saleswoman who you like and tell her you need some help picking out some new clothes to refresh your look. Let yourself relax and enjoy her attention! Seriously! Enjoy taking this time for yourself and having a new woman help you with your look! Give her a tip after completing your purchase! Be gracious and generous and act the part of being a gentleman. It feels good so let yourself enjoy it and give her appreciation for her help. Like your stylist she could become a great, fun friend and ally!

The clothes make the man, they say, and dressing the

part will lift your spirits and infuse your day with a more vibrant energy. Be sure to get new underwear too! Not just tidy whities briefs but try something different. Try some silk boxers, bamboo boy shorts or satin briefs! They feel amazing and are worth the expense. Why not treat yourself to some pleasure? Get some new shoes that look nice and are modern and cool too.

If you don't know where to start, then think of a man who you kind of idealize as a figure of male attractiveness and style. Then Google him and look at the image results and see what clothes he wears. Then go out and buy a couple outfits and accessories like shoes, belts, watches, hats, etc. that he would wear. It's fine to model your look after men whose appearance you like. It's a great starting point. It's not about pretending to be someone you're not-- it is about taking a little time and effort to care for yourself and your image. This self-care is seen and felt and speaks volumes to everyone around you. It makes you much more attractive. If you keep wearing the same clothes, you'll tend to keep acting the same way because how we look affects how we feel about ourselves.

What I'm saying here is that your definition of yourself is fluid, but fluids can stagnate! What we want here is to inject your life with some new energy by refreshing your look and giving you some new style and flair while at the same time giving you an infusion of female attention from outside of your relationship!

Even just a haircut and a new shirt will lift your spirits, but I challenge you to go further than that and give yourself the gift of an update to your look and some new female attention from a stylist and a saleswoman. Notice if the thought of receiving attention from other women causes you to feel fear or excitement or worry. Notice those feelings and then *let them be* and go out and do it regardless!

There's nothing wrong with having professional women help you in their area of professional expertise, so go and employ them to help you update your version of yourself. How many times do you do it in your life? Why not do it now? Remember: fuck your life! Enjoy it. Let yourself receive female attention. Even if it's hard, you can go do it! You're an adult. You'll enjoy the exchange of energy and you'll feel the benefits of it for a long time afterwards, and as a direct side benefit your partner will appreciate you taking care of yourself!

If any of this helped you or is hard for you, please go to the Facebook group (see the link in Appendix A) and share what you took away from this chapter or how people's energy towards you changed after doing a little style update! Make sure to keep up with your Kegel exercises and go out and update your style with the help of a couple of women!

Chapter 6: Hygiene

A foundational building block of intimacy is being clean and delicious. What are you serving your partner? I will be blunt here. Women like men who smell good. Good means a lot of things. It means "not bad" but it also means "not nothing." Good is a positive thing not a neutral thing. Not having any smell at all isn't "good," rather it's neutral-- an absence of smell. So, let me repeat myself: women like men who smell good. So, smell good! Yes, shower with soap daily, but that just makes you smell neutral. To smell good, you need to put something on that smells nice. Don't drown yourself in AXE like a high schooler or Old Spice like Grampa! Get something subtle and modern and understated that entices her and makes her want to come close to you to get a whiff. Think alluring. Think subtle... like she isn't sure that it's you that she's smelling.

Understand that many women are super sensitive to smells, so you don't want a powerful cologne. You want a subtle scent, and you may need to try a few different things before you find what she really likes. I recommend getting some natural essential oils like vetiver, cardamom, jasmine or cacao. Then just use a little bit every day and see how much she responds. Why not also go buy some all-natural dryer sheets and put them in the laundry to make your clothes smell fresh? Little things make a big difference. You want to intrigue her and capture her interest with her nose without overpowering her with harsh chemical scents. Her nose is a powerful way to either connect or repel. Use it to your advantage! We don't want to erase your scent entirely. We want scent honesty here, but we want to accent it while not being overpowering.

Now let's move on to your hands. Look at them. Look at your skin and nails. Look at your palms and fingerprints. Do you have long nails, sharp edges, calluses, hangnails, warts or cuts? Do the same with your feet. In order to be good at touching someone else we need to be more tuned in to our own experience of touch. A woman who wants a connection probably wants to be touched, and your hands are the most capable part of your body for touching her. Also, nobody likes dirty stinky calloused feet with long nails! Make your hands and feet soft so that you can touch her, and she won't feel like she's being scratched or sandpapered!

Use some coconut oil or Shea butter to soften your skin, and I recommend you get a nail clipper and just keep it on your keychain. Then whenever you are at work or driving and notice that you have long nails or hangnails, cut them back short. Also get a nail file and keep it with your toothbrush. If you ever get the chance to give your woman a yoni massage (a.k.a. a "hand job"), you'll *need* to have super short nails that are filed down smooth. Otherwise you run the risk of cutting her in her sensitive bits. If you have any calluses get an emery board and file them down regularly. While you are at it get some Shea butter cream or coconut oil and moisturize your hands once a day… especially before bed. Make your hands yummy, soft and delicious and she will love it when she feels how nice they are. If you have warts, do yourself and your lover a favor and Google a dermatologist in your area and make an appointment to get them treated. Ignoring them doesn't make them disappear, and they are contagious so it's the only respectful thing to do.

If you want her to enjoy kissing you, then think about the experience of your mouth for her. Of course, we must talk about your mouth and teeth. When was the last time you brushed or freshened your mouth? When was the last time you had a professional cleaning? Do you have visible plaque buildup on your teeth? Do you even know what plaque buildup looks like? What does your breath smell like? You must have nice breath! There are few things that are more of a turn-off to a woman than a man with bad breath, so get some mouthwash, and use it a few times a week to kill any built-up bacteria. Keep some floss on hand when you go out on your dates and check the mirror occasionally to make sure you don't have any food stuck in your teeth. And if your teeth are yellow from years of coffee or smoking, then getting them whitened at the dentist will give you a huge refresh and lease on life! It's a huge confidence booster.

Next let's check your hair. Women don't like sharp stubble, whether it's on your face or elsewhere on your body. Ask her what she likes the best: clean shaven face, ¼-inch long beard or longer beard. Ask her how she likes your pubic hair and body hair. Full length? Trimmed? Shaved daily? If you want her to enjoy your body, then think about making it as nice as possible for her to enjoy. Make sure to trim your nose and ear hairs weekly too. This isn't about being inauthentic. It's about being palatable and well groomed. The more you do it the better you will feel about yourself, and that comes across as confidence to everyone around you.

But we can't finish this chapter without talking about your penis and crotch and some unsavory stuff that can go on down there. Sorry if you think that this is obvious and doesn't need to be said, but I don't care. I'm going to say it anyway. Nobody wants to suck on a grungy cock that smells like piss and sweat with two days buildup of dead cells around the head. If you want your woman to go down on you (give you fellatio) and fuck your brains out, then you better make penis hygiene one of your top concerns because a clean cock has the best chance of getting some action.

Have you thoroughly checked your cock for warts recently? Examine it in good light and look for any small bumps or anything abnormal. If you are unsure then don't just sit in fear, but rather schedule a doctor's visit and get a professional opinion. Many little bumps on the skin of the penis and scrotum are normal little fatty deposits that help the skin to slide easily. Those are completely natural, normal and harmless, but if you are worried that they are an infection then go ask a doctor! If you have ever had a Sexually Transmitted Infection or been with someone who had an STI, then this is the time to do the right thing and go schedule a visit and get a checkup and STI test! It's a good thing to just get a comprehensive STI test once a year as a matter of practice for your own self-care because you never know if something was latent but then suddenly became contagious--even without symptoms! Please choose integrity in your actions when it comes to STIs, and your partners will learn that they can trust you because you demonstrate integrity.

If you have hemorrhoids or anything else like jock itch or a rash of any kind, then make an appointment to go get it checked out and addressed! If you have pimples on your butt or face or wherever, then go get some acne pads and start using them every day to clean the areas so that they start to dry up.

Take some pride in your skin and make it as enjoyable as possible. There's no better time than now. It's the largest organ of your body and the one that your woman wants to touch. Seriously. Do it for your sex life but also do it for your own health, because this is about you respecting yourself and taking care of yourself like a mature adult. No woman wants to have to mother her man like he's a child that can't take care of his own hygiene. Don't force her into seeing you as a boy rather than a man. If you want her to be able to be your hot lover, don't force her to act like a mother to you. Respect yourself and take care of *your* business. She'll see it and smell it and feel it and it'll make you significantly more attractive to her, and your confidence will make you a better human, man and lover.

Section 2:

Understand Your Partner

36

Chapter 7: Her Point of View

A mutually beneficial healthy relationship is built on trust and respect. If the foundation is good and strong then you can build a long-lasting relationship, but if the foundation isn't solid, the house will crumble eventually unless you put in a ton of work. It's much easier to build a solid foundation at the beginning than make repairs later!

I'm going to share with you what I believe to be perhaps the single biggest problem that men bring into their relationships with women. This is huge, and you might not like it. You might recoil and resist and deny it, but I've seen it over and over enough times to see how pervasive it is. So, open your mind, check your attitude at the door and let me say it to you straight.

Her point of view is no less valid than yours. Let me state it again. Her point of view is no less valid than yours.

Just let that sit there. Just let it sink in and notice if your mind reacts and immediately says some quick defensive judgments or opinions about it. It's interesting what comes up when you really sit with that statement.

Pretty much every man I know operates with an unspoken opinion that his point of view on the world is better, more right, and more valid than his partner's. It has to do with men thinking that "masculine" logical reasoning is more valid than "feminine" emotion and intuition. So many men will say that they believe that her point of view is just as valid as his, but when it really comes down to it, in the dirty nitty gritty of a long-term relationship, the ugly truth reveals itself. He often thinks that the way he sees things is the right way, and she is just being emotional or difficult.

She got along perfectly fine without you before, and if she suddenly had to live without you for the rest of her life, she would make it just fine. She'd make her money and get her bills paid and handle her needs just fine... and she'd do it her way.

When she says that she sees something one way notice if you interrupt her or feel or think that she's just wrong, and that if she could see it your way then she'd see that your way is obviously better because your way is based on logic. When you do that you put yourself on a high ground in your head and devalue her perspective, her wisdom, her experience, her insight and her intuition. If you interrupt her then you are just trying to make yourself right and make her wrong, and if you counter her statements and say things like, "Actually it's more X," or "You're wrong, it's Y," or "I wouldn't say it's that, actually it's Z," then pay particular attention here! It's much better to simply let her statement hang there in the air and then ask something like, "That's interesting. I don't see it that way, can you unpack that for me a little?" or "Huh, I never thought about it like that, can you explain that a bit more?"

The true power unfolds when the best of both worlds are brought to life and empowered by each other. Men accept her fully as your equal and then start letting her school you in her points of view. It will enrich your life. You will become more empathic and intuitive, and she will become more logical and organized as your experiences resonate with each other. You will improve each other and expand both of your skill sets and powers! All it takes is shining the light of reason on the tendency that you have, as a man, to think that your point of view is better than hers. Then destroy that belief by choosing to change it. Work up your courage and change something about yourself that will result in making you more able to meet a woman and empower her to embody herself fully in your presence.

Make it a practice. Whenever she says her opinion about something, just accept it as a valid opinion... just as valid as yours... and then if you don't completely agree with her ask her to tell you some more about why and how she sees it that way because that's not how you see it. If you experience a desire to set her straight or tell her how your idea is better, DON'T. Just DON'T. If you catch yourself interrupting, then apologize and ask her to continue.

Women have a term for men who tell them the way things are. They call it "mansplaining." It's a horribly derogatory term that I hate, but it exists because so many women have been talked over, talked down, dismissed, diminished and insulted by men thinking their point of view is more valid and wanting to be right more than wanting to have a successful connection.

Let her opinion float in your mind as a valid thought

stimulator and then try to see it from her perspective. Try to see how (from where she stands, and what she's gone through in life and the way that she thinks and has experienced things) her view makes sense and is logical from her perspective. Try counting to fifteen before you respond... and let yourself think during that time of different reasons why what she just said is true. Inherent in this practice you will find that you will come to value her perspective, and it will teach you things that you wouldn't learn if you just went around thinking you were right all the time.

If you really want to see things from her point of view when your instinct is to disagree, try saying, "You're right". Then immediately follow that up with a couple reasons that you come up with on the spot by feeling into what she's saying and letting your brain come up with a few rational reasons for why it's true from her perspective. You'll probably surprise yourself!

Let her enrich you. Don't sell your soul and not believe what you know to be true, but humble your ego and admit that you are not omnipotent. You are a product of your experiences and ideas and programming and limitations and failures and successes. A relationship with a woman can be the best thing in your life so let her expand your horizons and concepts, and you will be richer and wiser for it, and when you are authentically interested then she will *feel* your supporting recognition, your respect for her perspective, and it will fuel the fire between you.

Women respond well to men who empower and

respect them, so do this for yourself and for your relationship: Accept the truth that her point of view is just as valid as yours. Accept her as she is rather than requiring or wishing that she was different.

Chapter 8: Love Languages

One of the best ways to conceptualize the dynamic of love that I have ever come across is the metaphor of the love languages. This amazing way to look at love was developed by a relationship expert named Gary Chapman. After 30 years of working with couples he published a book called *The Five Love Languages*. The idea is that different people feel loved in different ways, and what works for one person may not work for another. He calls these "love languages." They are: 1) words of affirmation, 2) quality time, 3) receiving gifts, 4) acts of service, and 5) physical touch. While each of us can enjoy each of these ways to feel love, most of us respond most strongly to one or two of them.

If you don't know what language your love language is, and if you don't know in which way you can really feel loved then you are not empowered to ever be successful in being loved! You simply won't know what your love needs are, so you won't be able to get them met! Words are power. They define thoughts and concepts. So, if you don't have a word... a phrase... a name for a concept, then you are prevented from being able to focus your mental powers on it and overcome its challenges.

So, let's go over them one by one, and then I'll give you a quick way to determine what your primary love language is.

1. **Words of affirmation**. Mark Twain once said, "I can live for two months on a good compliment." This is totally true to people who respond to words of affirmation. If you need to hear compliments, verbal encouragement, kind words or humble words in order to feel loved then learn this term: "words of affirmation," and start thinking about how words and the feelings they invoke are important to you. Lots of men have a deep need for verbal appreciation for the work they do to support their partner and family. If that resonates with you then understand that you need words of affirmation to feel loved. Then you can communicate it to your partner, thereby giving her the tools to love you in the way that you need to be loved in order to feel loved.

2. **Quality time**. Some people really need to have focused attention from their partner in order to feel loved. You know: time alone without distraction or responsibility on your shoulders where you can really enjoy being together. It's where you have each other's undivided attention with quality conversation and doing quality activities together just because you love being together. Quality time is a way to express love, and if you need this from your partner then learn the term so that you can own it and communicate it to her.

3. **Receiving gifts.** This is a universal trait of love around the world. Everywhere on the planet people in love give gifts to each other to show their love. To some people it's important to receive gifts, but to other people it's not so important. If this is your love

43

language, then receiving gifts from your partner is essential for you feeling like she loves you. They can be physical or symbolic, inexpensive or expensive. Most importantly the act of giving is a visible and tangible demonstration of love that some people absolutely need to receive from their partners.

4. **Acts of Service**. This is basically doing things that you know your partner would like for you to do for her. It's pleasing your partner by serving her and expressing love by doing things for her. Things like cooking dinner, cleaning the house, paying the bills, walking the dog, etc.... are all acts of service. They require thought and planning and time to accomplish and must be done with a free and positive spirit to be meaningful. These can be requested, but they can't be demanded or else it will stop the feeling of love in them.

5. **Physical Touch**. Holding hands, kissing, shoulder rubs, sex, hugs, tickles, wrestling, massage, dancing... these are all forms of physical touch, and some people really need it in order to feel loved. Other people simply don't, but if you need to be touched in order to feel loved, you'll know it--and lack of it can be a deal breaker for you! Ask and communicate--because the kind of touch that feels good to you may not feel good to her--so it needs to be investigated and understood. Too much touch or bad touch can clearly be abuse, so it must be done lovingly and consciously.

Now that you know that there are love languages go figure out what your love language is. It'll only take a few minutes, but once you are done then you'll know exactly how you need to be shown love in order to feel loved, and then you can take that information forward into your life and own it... discuss it with your partner and craft your life so that you get more of what you need. Now, it's possible to have two love languages or even a mix of three that are your primary ones and doing this exercise will show you that.

Go to Appendix C at the back of this book and fill out the worksheet to discover your primary love language. I recommend you copy the worksheet and have your partner fill it out to find out what her primary love language is also. That will empower you to love her the way that she needs to be loved for her to *feel* loved by you!

Once you both know your love languages, a whole new world will open to you where your love for each other can be received by each other. It's a huge tool, and I encourage you to go buy the book *The Five Love Languages* and read it together.

Ok you awesome relationship-preneur. That's all for this chapter. Remember to keep up with your Kegels and to fuck your life every day, and if you have any questions or comments please post them in the Facebook group (see Appendix A at the back of this book for the link).

Chapter 9: Female Arousal Roadmap

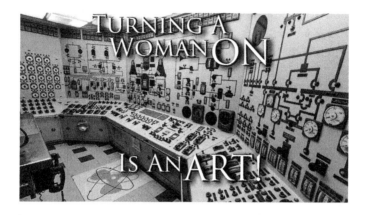

I've not found anything hotter than an emboldened woman who is thoroughly aroused, unashamed and feeling like a sexual Goddess. Women can be tricky to arouse compared to men however, but if you understand the roadmap then you can get there with a little effort. Let me tell you that it is worth the work to learn this roadmap!

Most men make lots of mistakes when trying to please a woman. They don't pay attention to her subtle cues, body language, breath and tone. They are clumsy or rough or abrasive with their touch and attitude, and they go for her genitals and for penetration *way too fast* while ignoring all the delicious lusciousness of her body and the mood and the emotional high... basically not enjoying the journey and just rushing to the destination.

Let's use a metaphor here. Generalizations are often

problematic, but I find them to be a useful teaching tool here even though there are always exceptions. That said, let's say that feminine energy, also known as Yin energy, is watery and cool and slow to heat up. It is like a fluid, and it can be easily blocked. Masculine energy, also known as Yang energy, is fiery and hot and fast to burn. For both of your pleasure it is better for you to slow down... cool down to match her speed and temperature than it is for you to want her to heat up and speed up to a quick burn out. Quickies are great, don't get me wrong, but we're talking about the bigger context of how female arousal works overall and how to work with it for the benefit of your relationship.

If what you want is for your female partner to be a sex goddess, if you really want her to fucking love sex with you and be totally wild and free and playful and orgasmic and to have transcendent sex with you with a chance at having a spiritual or divine connection and exquisite ecstasy--then you need to understand how she works. Women are often taught to play small and keep their sexual power in a box. You have the lucky possibility of being the key to unlock that box by creating a safe space where she can really open up and share herself deeply—both sexually and emotionally. I find a top-down metaphor works great here.

First: start at her head, her mind, her crown chakra. The brain is the most powerful erogenous zone that a woman has! You can connect to her mentally with conversation, showing her that you respect her intelligence, exploring sexy ideas and fantasies with her, teasing her intellect and getting her to think about things that are arousing. In general women like conversation, so don't be the dull bump on a log who never asks her about her day or how she's feeling or what's happening inside of her! Be interested in her and engage in conversation with her about things that are on her mind and about things that you've been thinking about. If you aren't engaged with her mind, she probably won't be able to engage deeply with you with her body.

Moving lower with our top down metaphor to her heart: give her what her heart needs. Women's hearts need connection to warm up. They need to talk and touch and listen and share. They need to feel loved. They need to feel your attention and presence with her emotionally in order to create the context of emotional rapport and affinity that causes her heart to open. This is done by action more than conversation. How does she experience love? Did you do the Love Languages exercise with her? Love her in the way that she experiences love, whether that is gifts, acts of service, words of affirmation, quality time or physical touch. To connect to her heart, I recommend you love her daily *in her primary love language*.

Then move lower still: to her gut, where instinctive reactions take place and shame resides. She needs to feel safe and secure. She needs reassurance from you. She needs to feel like you have addressed the things that can get in the way of her arousal. Kids, dirty dishes, bills, health issues, past trauma, her feelings about her body, her fears. All these instinctual gut reactions can block her feminine energy from flowing further down to her root chakra at her sex and heating up her genitals, but if you address the concerns and fears and reassure her congruently then the energy can flow freely through her gut and on down to warm her up at her root. So do the dishes and put the kids to sleep and pay the bills and tell her that you are going to do them all so that they are done --and so that she can relax a bit. If you aren't sure what she's worried about or what things might get in the way of her feeling sexy, then just ask her directly, "Hey, honey, I want to help you to be able to relax, so I want to ask you what things are on your mind lately that I could help with?"

This is just one way to think about turning on a woman. From her mind to her heart to her gut to her genitals. And if you get the energy flowing freely from the top down, *then* you can arouse her genitals with physical touch and penetration, and she can respond into becoming the juicy sex goddess who you want to play with. You must give her what she wants from you though. She wants you to be focused on her, and to demonstrate that you are dedicated and devoted to her pleasure, that you are clear with your intentions and are into integrity--not manipulating or lying.

What I mean is that you must *demonstrate* to her that you have integrity, not just telling her. Doing what you say you will do, saying what you mean and meaning what you say, being reliably, honest and transparent demonstrates integrity. Know what you want and speak it clearly and honestly. Let her know that you want her, that you love her body, what parts you love about her body and why. Do you like the way she looks, smells, tastes? Share that with her.

49

Explain how and why she's yummy to you. It reassures her, if you do it honestly and are consistent, but if you aren't congruent you can't fake it and expect success.

That said, listen: if you don't take anything else away from this but this one single thing, don't go for her genitals or try to penetrate her until she is completely turned on and hot from crown to root. In other words, wait until she's absolutely craving you to be inside of her! Anything other than that and she isn't completely ready, and you won't be truly welcome into the temple, and without that you'll never get to meet the sex goddess who is waiting inside.

Now, I'm not talking about consent here. We'll get to that. What I'm talking about is understanding the female roadmap to arousal, i.e. how women get turned on. Understanding this metaphor doesn't mean you'll get a green light all the time, but rather it gives you a deeper understanding of the terrain so that you can navigate better and therefore will have higher chances of successful pleasurable experiences together!

While of course you could just dive into the deep end and go for her genitals right away and have a quickie--let me ask you, how fun would every movie be if they only lasted 5 minutes?

Chapter 10: Setting

One of the biggest inhibitors to sex and intimacy that women experience is too much worry, concern and distraction. If she has a lot on her mind or on her shoulders, or if she's always nervous that someone is going to walk in on you, then she's never going to be able to relax. The set and setting of your home and lovemaking space are tangible physical things that probably affect her ability and desire to be sexy with you.

Think about the room where you can have sex with your partner. Is it beautiful, yummy and inviting? Is it messy with stuff all over the place? Is it private? Can she ever really relax there? How is the bed? Is it super comfy, or is it a crappy 30-year-old mattress? Think like a lover. To facilitate having an amazing sex life with your partner you need to create and foster a safe and clean place where both of you can relax in privacy and let go of your inhibitions and worries. Don't just buy new sheets but put them on the bed too! Don't just do the laundry but put it away too! A bottle of spray cleaner and a roll of paper towels could transform your space for her enjoyment and yours!

Even if you can't "fix it" make it better by doing some improvements. It's very off-putting for a woman to see her lover put zero effort or care into making the bedroom a place of physical comfort. You see women often think or feel that if you can't even take care of your bedroom then how attentive of a lover will you be? Clean up the room at least, or maybe go buy some new pillows or wash the curtains and get some incense or essential oil diffuser to make the room smell better. If it smells like cats or dogs or kids, it won't help you have a sexy time together. Just covering up a bad smell with perfume isn't going to help. Washing the stinky stuff is more important than spraying the room with perfume! Is the light too bright and abrasive? Get a lamp with a dimmer and a shade. Do you have a stereo in the room that you can play some relaxing sexy music on? If not, then set one up. Can the neighbors see in the windows? Does the door have a good lock to keep the kids out? The idea is to create a safe place for you both to feel secure enough to get intimate together where you won't be disturbed.

If you can't do much to improve the bedroom because of real-world things like kids, pets, neighbors, family, etc., then shift your focus and go find a motel or hotel or bed & breakfast nearby that will work. Go on your own and check a few out. Ask to see the rooms. Smell them with your nose when you walk in. Check if there is a bathtub. Is there good hot water? Sit on the bed. Is it yummy? Does it squeak when you wiggle? Find a place that is the best and most inviting and luxurious place that you can find and afford occasionally that is close by and put their number into your phone. Then use it! Don't wait for it to be the perfect night. If you can find a few hours in the middle of the day or the week when you can be alone together, then go rent the room and use it for some quality time alone.

This is just one example of a concern that might be an inhibitor to her being able to relax. If your bedroom is a cluttered space that isn't very private, it won't facilitate relaxation and connection. If it's a joyous place of rejuvenation, relaxation and sensual delights then it will help to encourage the two of you getting into your physical sensual bodies together. Ask your lover what she likes in the environment. What music does she enjoy? Does she prefer silence? Does she prefer candlelight? What scents? Does she prefer to make love in the morning, daytime or nighttime? Learn her likes so you can use them to love her better!

Identify distractions for her and address them or get rid of them! Look at your bedroom and bathroom and clean them up, and then do three things in each of them to make them more yummy and inviting. Make it lovely and make it a safe-space for the two of you to be intimate together! You'll both appreciate it, and it will give you a physical place to foster your emotional connection.

Chapter 11: Barriers to Intimacy

I know that many men can be in the mood to have sex almost anywhere and anytime or everywhere and every time. Women are different and if you take steps to understand them, you'll be better able to interface with her, support her and foster a situation in which she might be able to relax and be open to you.

For most women, worries on their minds, weights on their shoulders and concerns that tighten their gut are all things that are poisonous to their arousal. After a stressful day with loud kids, a traffic jam and some bills that are overdue, sex with you is probably the last thing on her mind! You need to understand that. If you force it, you'll just show that you are a jerk.

If you want to improve your relationship and your sex life, then you need to learn how to work with her and help her when she is worried, stressed, concerned or overwhelmed. Don't add to her list of problems by being pushy or not-understanding. You need to learn to listen to her and not tell her how to fix things. You have a choice. You can either be part of the problem or part of the solution. It's better for your relationship and your sex life if you are part of the solution.

What we are talking about here is opening your eyes and reading her, seeing where she is at, feeling what she's dealing with and then connecting with her right in the middle of it all. You are demonstrating your caring here.

Look at her and listen to her and think about her. What is she stressed out about and bothered by? What's been really nagging at her lately? Figure it out if you can and if you can't then simply ask her what's bothering her and going on for her. Tell her you want to know because you want to connect with her--where she's at! If you are going to remove inhibitors to intimacy, then you need to find out what's weighing her down.

Then when you find out what those things are, address them. You don't have to fix them! She may not want you to anyway. Don't just be a jerk and tell her how she should fix it. Rather, acknowledge the issues and try to understand how they make her feel. Feel some empathy. If it's something you can support her with, then tell her you would like to help her with it, if she would like your help.

You don't have to solve the problem, but if you can demonstrate that you are honestly concerned and committed to helping reduce the problem and have a plan then she may be able to lay down her worry and concern about that issue for a while. We're talking about connecting with her and becoming her ally with addressing the things that bring her down, without taking over and without just trying to fix it with a judgment or quick solution. Instead of offering solutions just say, "I see this is getting to you, is there anything I can do to support you?" Then listen to what she says *carefully*.

If she's stressed because she's tired and the house is a mess, then those are real things that you can do to help make her feel better: make dinner and clean up the house!

If she's stressed because you are in a mountain of debt then talk about it and say you are stressed about it too and that you want to make a plan to make it better so that you can still connect with each other in the meantime and work together to make a better future.

Doing these things doesn't mean that you are absolutely going to succeed in getting her in the mood to have sex with you, but I guarantee you that it will help her to feel better, and she'll appreciate it. If anything will help you to get her interested in having sex with you it will be her appreciating you and feeling like you support her where she is at without requiring her to be different than she is. Being her ally, finding where she is at and then meeting her there and demonstrating your loving willingness to help her with her burdens... that fosters connection, which is the root of female sexual desire. When you can name and address each worry one by one... you effectively reduce their power at inhibiting her being able to relax into the sensual connective part of her being. This is why dates and vacations are so important. You get out of the house, away from all the usual problems, and get to relax and let go of your regular worries for a little while.

Tracking and gauging your partner's mental and emotional landscape is a beautiful practice to get into and if she feels you tracking her thoughts and emotions and demonstrating that you care about them, it will demonstrate that you care about her, and women respond to tangible real proof that you care!

So, go out and start knocking out any intimacy inhibitors that you can identify and connect with your partner because you love her and want to be close to her!

Chapter 12: Her Monthly Cycle

I'm going to share with you a tool to really empower you to improve how you can support and connect to your partner. It's simple. It's fast. It's free, and you use it on your phone.

A few years ago, I realized that I really needed to keep track of my partner's monthly cycle. Her changes would often completely take me by surprise, and I wanted to be empowered rather than bewildered. So, I downloaded a few apps that women use to track their menstrual cycles and I tried them out.

What a good idea that turned out to be!

Now of course every woman is different, and if your partner is peri-menopausal or has gone through menopause then this advice won't apply, but if she is in her fertile "child-rearing" years then you can get a lot of benefit from this lesson.

Whether you know it or not there are two distinct emotional periods that many women go through each month as their hormone levels regularly change. If you learn these periods and what happens for your partner in each of them, then you can be equipped to handle and support and even enjoy them as they happen--turning the tables on them and using them to empower and support your relationship rather than bring chaos and cause misunderstanding between you.

It's the path of a conscious lover to love all of her, not just the parts that you enjoy. I mean this both in terms of her personality and emotions, and also her body and its changes. If you can learn to love all the aspects of her that occur in her life, she will learn that she can count on you and that she won't have to hide from you. When she feels that she can lean into you and trust you to take the true weight of the honest reality of her, then she can relax into areas of mental, emotional, sexual and erotic exploration with you that maybe she's never done with anyone in her life ever before.

UNDERSTANDING THE CYCLE EMPOWERS YOUR RELATIONSHIP!

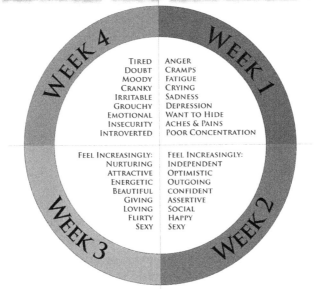

WEEK 4

WEEK 1

TIRED	ANGER
DOUBT	CRAMPS
MOODY	FATIGUE
CRANKY	CRYING
IRRITABLE	SADNESS
GROUCHY	DEPRESSION
EMOTIONAL	WANT TO HIDE
INSECURITY	ACHES & PAINS
INTROVERTED	POOR CONCENTRATION

FEEL INCREASINGLY:	FEEL INCREASINGLY:
NURTURING	INDEPENDENT
ATTRACTIVE	OPTIMISTIC
ENERGETIC	OUTGOING
BEAUTIFUL	CONFIDENT
GIVING	ASSERTIVE
LOVING	SOCIAL
FLIRTY	HAPPY
SEXY	SEXY

WEEK 3

WEEK 2

I've made a quick little pie chart that gives a grossly over generalized summary of the periods. Use it as a general road map, but don't take is as universal fact! Each woman is completely unique, and it is much more important to learn your partner's specific cycle than the gross generalizations that I put in this chart.

That said, this is still a good place to start from research I've compiled by women on women. Find out when she starts her period, and that is the beginning of week number one. Then you can map out into the future when the best times and worst times will be to do certain things. For example, don't plan a dance date for when she's going to be having cramps and feeling like she wants to hide away from the world. Do plan an awesome vacation for the week that she's probably going to be feeling outgoing and playful. The idea is to work with her cycles to empower your life together, and when you know that she's likely to be feeling indrawn, introspective, tired and sensitive, then you can be extra nice and caring and supportive or give her the distance that she may desire. She'll love you the more for it and you will both get along better for it because you will know her better and how to interface with her consciously.

Here's a quick rough summary: The two main hormones involved in a woman's cycle are estrogen and progesterone (see chart below). Estrogen is a hormone that makes people feel good and happy while progesterone is considered a "stress" chemical that causes depression. Every month a woman experiences her body cycling between being high on happy hormones and then having her prescription changed without her consent to a depressant for the next two weeks. Imagine what that would be like for you if you were force fed mood enhancers for two weeks then depressants for the following two weeks, for your entire adult life!

Of course, every woman is different, and some may feel this severely while others may not notice this at all. Also, any single woman's experience of her monthly cycle changes over time. Generally however, the effects of these two hormones have been proven and their densities in the bloodstream have been measured and charted to reveal a regular pattern.

As shown in the chart below, you will see that for week one and two her estrogen levels slowly build, generally causing her to feel increasingly optimistic and outgoing, happy, confident, and social. She may be sharp and clear, relatively unstressed and less sensitive to pain and discomfort. These generally are the great weeks to plan activities with other people, vacations and dates, and she may generally feel playful, fun and sexier day-by-day right up until the estrogen peaks on the day she ovulates. So, if you want to plan for a time when you might have a fun, hot and erotic time together then plan to have a romantic date around her ovulation day. Women can be excited about lovemaking when they are ovulating so be ready to really show up and show some stamina if you awaken her erotic potentials during this time!

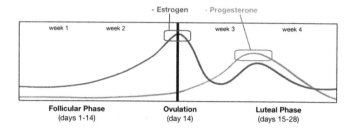

- Estrogen   - Progesterone

| week 1 | week 2 | week 3 | week 4 |

| Follicular Phase | Ovulation | Luteal Phase |
| (days 1-14) | (day 14) | (days 15-28) |

Be conscious that making love when she is ovulating also carries the highest risk of pregnancy, so remember to address that concern in order to remove it as a mental barrier to intimacy. Whether it means getting and using condoms (or some other form of birth control) or not having intercourse and instead doing only other forms of sexual lovemaking (cunnilingus, yoni massage, anal sex, etc.), be an ally and take the necessary steps so that you both can relax fully into the erotic deliciousness because you've addressed the pregnancy concern!

After she ovulates, she may experience an estrogen crash quickly followed by a rise in the stress hormone progesterone which often causes a person to feel depressed, increasingly irritable, sensitive, emotional, moody, stressed and hungry. She might become introverted, intuitive, sad, or have sudden mood swings and become more sensitive to annoyances, pain and discomfort. This is when you want to shine in your capacity to provide loving support and kindness to her. Take the opportunity to show her that you care by doing things to help her feel loved and cared for. A hot water bottle and hot soup when she has cramps goes a long way to demonstrate that you understand and care for her, and being able to "read her" and meet her in the middle of her experience demonstrates that you care deeply for her.

There is a lot of information out there to help you understand the hormonal basis for these time periods and to more precisely map your partner's recurring circular tendencies so go read them! I highly recommend mymoontime.com for information, and I personally use the Clue and myFlo apps on my phone.

Although it shouldn't need to be said, *never* tell her she's being emotional or irrational! Doing that just shows that you don't understand her and aren't strong enough to handle her powerful feminine energy! If she is experiencing emotional ping pong and it is exhausting for you then it is best to just show her that you love her and support her. Give her space but be close by if she needs you, and when she does then *be* there with your attention and presence and be ready to be real with her. She might just let you hold her in a moment of intensity in which she's never let anyone else in! These are keys to the sacred realm here, brothers. Wield this power with proper high intention and conscious love and it will bring you together and she will love you more for it, and you will love her more as you come to see and understand her more deeply for the amazing being that she is.

One of my female friends told me, "Most men don't know that every month they have a relationship with two different women." I don't quite agree with her, but it is a fun thought stimulator to think of when considering the competing effects of estrogen and progesterone. So, go download Clue or some other period tracking app and check out mymoontime.com, and get a clue about your partner's cycle and start using it to empower and connect the two of you!

Section 3:

Increase Your Sex Education

Chapter 13: Birth Control

Let's talk about birth control. It's a multi-faceted issue that really can inhibit you having a toe curlingly juicy sex life with your partner, unless you both are trying to get pregnant. But if a pregnancy isn't something you both want right now then the fear of pregnancy can really get in the way of her relaxing into deep sexual arousal and responsiveness to your desires, and on the other hand if she ends up getting pregnant then that will *really* kill your sex life and weigh you both down with thoughts, fears and decisions that will smother the fire that you want to kindle here.

For way too long men have considered it the woman's problem to protect herself from getting pregnant, but that's the old male-chauvinistic way. What we are doing here is learning how to bridge the gap between the sexes in order to foster profound intimacy. To do that men have to stand up and take responsibility for our actions and their repercussions. No woman wants to be knocked up by a man who doesn't want to be the father of her child, and no man wants to raise a child that he doesn't want, and then there's child support and of course a beautiful new child that comes into the world - in yet another broken home with fighting parents.

Enough of that already!

Men, take responsibility for the fact that your cum is a pregnancy producing army! Don't go putting that stuff up where babies come from unless you want to make a baby or have taken steps to address it! I'm advocating that you take responsibility for your pregnancy producing potential here rather than relying on her. Why put such an important decision into the hands of another? It's your life force, after all!

You have three main options available to you today. Pick one and *use it!*

1) If you know you never want to have children then go get a vasectomy. The procedure can cost anywhere from free to $500, is very minor surgery, and has an almost 100% birth control success rate these days. The benefits of this are stunningly profound. It changes the experience of your ejaculation for the woman. No longer is your cum something that is to be feared and guarded against. No longer is it a threat. It becomes a delicious fluid that can be deliciously enjoyed. It's truly amazing to have your life essence be craved by your partner rather than disliked and shunned.

2) If you might want to have children in the future but not now, then you can still go get a vasectomy but do it *after* you go save some sperm at a fertility clinic for future use. You go to the fertility clinic, make your deposits and they freeze them and save them. They are good for 20 years or more! Then when you decide that you want to have children you and your partner go to the clinic, they monitor her fertility and then at the perfect moment deposit the thawed sperm in the exact right location for her to conceive. There is a yearly

storage cost, and then the cost of the insemination procedure can be in the range of $500 to $1,000. It's a small cost when compared to the cost of an abortion or the emotional cost of an unwanted pregnancy. After making your deposits then go get your vasectomy and then you can have permanent birth control (ahh… yes… relax!!!) *and* can still have children, but only when you decide you want to! It's a game-changer.

3) If you can't do that then the cheapest and second-best method that I recommend is to carry condoms and *use them* every time you have vaginal intercourse, and get a monthly menstrual cycle app on your phone like the one I use, Clue, and track your partner's fertility cycle. Then when she's in her fertile window, *don't* have vaginal intercourse at all--not even with a condom. Consider choosing to not ejaculate at all, or ask her if she'd like you to come somewhere else. Does she like it on her boobs or belly or in her mouth or in her ass or on her butt or nowhere at all? The only way to know and be respectful is to ask. Wherever you release, just don't deposit your little baby making army up anywhere near her love canal! Even coming on her pussy lips can get her pregnant so be conscious, be aware and put it somewhere else. A lot of people around the world use anal sex during the fertility period to avoid pregnancy, and it's a decent measure if she enjoys anal sex and likes doing it with you, but the only ethical way to know is to ask her and not pressure her (see Appendix E). If you aren't sure how to bring it up, then read Chapter 25 and check out Appendix B

where there is a worksheet on how to bring up a difficult topic.

Now if you choose to use condoms, understand that they are only about 80% to 90% effective when used perfectly, which means that out of 100 couples using condoms 10 to 20 will get pregnant in a year of absolutely perfect condom use.

The reality however is that condoms slip off and break sometimes. As a result actual real-world pregnancy rates are significantly higher. Statistically around 20 to 30 out of every 100 couples get pregnant each year with condom use. Note that that's each year. So if you choose condoms as your birth control method for a multi-year relationship you have about a 25% chance of getting pregnant in year one, a 25% chance in year two, 25% in year three and 25% in year four. It's hypothetically 100% certain that you'll get pregnant within four years of real-world condom use because the chances can be seen as cumulative year by year.

You don't want to cause an unwanted pregnancy--so if you are going to only use condoms, use a period tracking app, avoid vaginal intercourse during her fertile window, and make sure that you get condoms that fit tightly enough to not slip off. Most major brands have "slim" or "thin" condoms that are a little tighter to help them not slip off. Also make sure that your condom is in perfect condition and hasn't expired. Carrying them in your wallet for a long time makes them weak, as well as if they are exposed to heat or cold like leaving them in your car during the summer or winter.

The spermicide in spermicidal condoms can often cause irritation for you and your partner, and that irritation decreases the condoms' effectiveness at protecting against STIs, so I don't recommend spermicidal condoms. Again, my recommendation here is to get a vasectomy. However, if you can't do that it's an excellent strategy to aim for perfect condom use with a conscious choice not to ejaculate inside or near her vagina around her fertile window because you are tracking her cycle.

Remember, worrying about pregnancy can get in the way of a woman relaxing into a juicy sexfest with you. Recognize the elephant in the room and decide for yourself to make a plan and stick to it. She'll respect and appreciate you for it as you show her that you respect and value her. Once you've addressed the issue then you both get to relax that part of your mind and slip into the yummy sexual deliciousness that you really want to have with each other.

Chapter 14:
Sexually Transmitted Infections

Most people hate to talk about it, but if you want to empower your sex life then we have to talk about sexually transmitted infections. We used to call them STDs but with all the advances in treatment and understanding now we call them STIs because there is always treatment available for an infection and calling them diseases was incorrect.

Nowadays there are over ten common STIs that are going around, and there are many smaller lesser known ones that don't make the top ten list. There's hepatitis B and hepatitis C, chlamydia, HIV and AIDS, gonorrhea, syphilis, herpes, scabies, fungus, pubic lice, warts (aka HPV), molloscum contagiosum, nongonococcal urethritis (aka NGU) and cytomegalovirus (aka CMV), and those are just the main ones!

STIs have a lot of stigma and carry a lot of shame, but just like colds, flus and skin conditions like eczema, shingles, chicken pox, and jock itch, they can be thought of as normal human infections that don't deserve to be seen as shameful. Redefining the meaning that we give them is very important because it frees us up to talk about them without it being so heavy. Sex is natural. Sicknesses are natural. They both happen. You aren't a bad person because you caught a cold, nor are you a bad person if you catch a virus! Think about someone you love who has become sick. You don't think badly of them because they became ill, do you? If you let go of the instilled programming that makes you think that STIs are inherently "dirty" then you can think of someone with an STI with just as much kindness as you would think of someone with cancer.

If you have ever had sex with anyone and if you ever plan or hope to have sex with anyone in the future, then you owe it to yourself to learn a little bit about STIs so that you will be as healthy and happy in your life as possible! With overpopulation and increasing population density, STIs are spreading and mutating faster than ever before.

I know it's not sexy and it's not fun, but what we are doing here is redefining our relationship with sex and empowering our lives through knowledge and communication.

A lot of people think that since they know how one STI is transmitted and what it does to the body they know about all of them, and that is a terribly dangerous mistake to believe. Each of the STIs acts differently, is spread differently, and affects a different area of the body. Knowing about one does not mean you know about them all!

Do you think you are STI-free because you have no symptoms? Think again. Do you think it's okay to have sex without a condom because your partner doesn't have any symptoms of an STI? Not so fast. The truth is that usually STIs don't show symptoms. They can lay dormant for years *while remaining contagious* and then can cause problems later.

So, let's take a minute and go over the main types. There are skin to skin contact transmission STIs and there are STIs that are transmitted through bodily fluids. Condoms and gloves are great at protecting against the STIs that are spread by bodily fluids when used correctly during penetrative sex, but they don't protect against skin to skin transmission on areas of skin not covered by them.

Many times an STI can infect a person and not show symptoms because they are healthy, but it can still be transmitted. Then if they ever get sick or have a suppressed immune system the STI can flare up and surprise them. For a lot of people who experience an STI they may never know when or by whom they were infected, and it's a horrible feeling to be sick, let alone the fact that it can make you feel dirty and full of shame because there is so much negative stigma about sex in our culture. It's not something you want, and it's worth protecting yourself even if you already have one or two STIs. I guarantee you that you don't want more!

Getting tested is something that everyone who is sexually active or plans to be sexually active should do. Usually you just need a physical exam, a conversation with a doctor and to pee in a cup. Sometimes you might need to get swabbed or to have blood drawn. It's quick and worth its weight in gold because knowledge is power. If you find out you have an STI then you can get it treated! Take action! Don't just sit there in ignorance because you are afraid of what you might learn. You owe it to yourself to take care of your body's health. It's the only body you'll ever have, and you want it to last a long time!

Even if you are in a monogamous long-term relationship you should still go get tested. Even if you both thought you were disease-free when you got together and still think you are STI-free now, something could have been dormant inside you. What if your partner has HPV and doesn't know it? HPV, human papillomavirus, can cause cancer and is often symptom-free. They could give it to you, and if you don't have it yet it doesn't mean that you couldn't get it in the future. You'd want them to protect you, wouldn't you? Well, you should do the same for them.

If you are dating or having sex with multiple people, then it's even more important. Go get tested now so you know. Then use condoms and get tested every half year or year.

I've noticed that a lot of people with a high tolerance for risk tend to minimize their sense of potential consequences and have a "never happen to me" mentality. But when it comes to STIs that mentality isn't worth a damn. *Anyone* can get an STI, and the only responsible way to deal with it is to get tested, communicate any infections to your partners, and ask them to get tested and communicate any infections they have with you.

Having an STI doesn't have to be a deal breaker, but it's better to know. Many STIs can be addressed by simply wearing a condom and not sharing any bodily fluids. That means no ejaculating in her vagina, ass, mouth or on her face (because your semen could get in her eyes or nose or mouth). But there's plenty that you can do with your hands and with condoms on. Men, if your partner asks or requires you to wear a condom then be honorable and do it. Don't pressure her not to use one, and don't slip it off when she won't notice. It's a really disgusting thing to do and it would only prove that you have no honor, no credibility to your word, and that you can't be trusted. At worst it'll land you in jail and define you as a sex offender and sexual predator as well as a male supremacist. What we are doing here is raising our vibration to become conscious lovers, and the benefits of that are that women will respond more to you and want to share themselves deeper than ever before.

If you find out that you have an STI, then do the honorable thing and communicate it to your partner and all past partners. Because there is so much shame and stigma around this you may be afraid of doing it. I understand. It could be terrifying. The good news is that there's a way to not let that stop you. There are services available that let you tell your partners anonymously. That way you are being ethical about communicating the essential information, but you avoid having to receive judgment, blame and shame. See the recommended resources section in Appendix A at the back of this book for a link to one of these anonymous notification services.

Let me tell you that if you both get tested and both turn out to be STI-free, then you can relax into sharing your sexual juices and bodies together freely. It is the most profound deliciousness to be able to relax your brain and put down your worries about STIs and just play and delight in each other's sexual parts and liquids.

Your homework is to go schedule an appointment to get tested and to read up on the various common STIs, their means of transmission and how to prevent them! Make some decisions for yourself about what your safer sex boundaries and requirements are considering the different common STIs and get yourself a safer sex kit.

Chapter 15: Lubricants

This is a power course on lubes to supercharge your understanding so that you can make your sex life better than ever. Most people think that there's not much to know about lubes. You just pick something slippery and it helps, right? Wrong!

Using the wrong thing can cause lots of problems including infections and hindering pregnancy (which is a concern if you want to conceive). In my professional opinion the single best lube for sex is a woman's natural lubrication. As a general rule of thumb (with exceptions of course), if you aren't getting her hot enough to be wet enough to have intercourse with you then she isn't ready for intercourse! That said, some women can't get sufficiently wet no matter how aroused they are because of their unique biology and health status, and also some women are wet all the time—even if they aren't aroused! The safest way to know her level of arousal is to get to know your partner intimately. Ask her about her experience of her natural lubrication and its relationship to her arousal. In the absence of her saying that she can't get wet or is always wet, it's safer for you to use her lubrication level as an indicator of her arousal than to assume that she's ready for intercourse when she isn't wet!

I see it as nature's built-in elegant feedback mechanism, and it can guide you to become a better lover. Unless she's told you (or you've observed) that this rule doesn't apply to her, if she isn't dripping wet and craving you to fill her yet then my advice is don't enter her yet. Focus on heating her to the boiling point where she can't take it any longer and just needs to have you inside her already! It's the key to being a kickass lover, and it can help turn her into a ravenous sex goddess.

However there are plenty of situations when this advice doesn't apply at all. For example: if the guy's cock is huge and uncomfortable for the woman, or if you are going to have anal sex, or if she has a physiological issue that prevents her from producing sufficient lubrication regardless of her level of arousal, or if you want to have great sex in the shower or hot tub where her natural lubrication gets washed away by the water.

For all those situations I want to share with you the dangers and implications of various common lubes. There are natural lubes, synthetic lubes, petroleum-based lubes, oil-based, water-based, and silicone-based lubes, and then there are all kinds of gimmick lubes to increase sensation through heat or cooling, reduce sensation by numbing, and flavored and scented and even glow in the dark lubes! That said, the vagina will absorb into her bloodstream anything that you put into it so it's extremely important to not put anything unhealthy or full of chemicals or toxins in it.

First let's cover the basics of all manufactured lubes. You see, the natural pH level of the vagina is slightly acidic. Manufactured personal lubricants are designed to be acidic to mimic this. This is bad if you are trying to conceive a child as the lube will enhance the overall acidity of the vagina and make it harder to get pregnant. For conception it's best to use just the woman's natural lubrication, but if you must have an auxiliary lube then get one like Yes Baby Fertility Friendly Lube. It mimics the pH balance and osmolarity of semen and is best during ovulation.

Now the most common and well-known type of lube is water-based lube like Astroglide or K-Y Jelly, although I don't recommend those exact two because they contain an antiseptic-like ingredient that is bad for the vagina. In general however, water-based lubes are easy to clean up with soap and water and are really slick initially. They are easy to find and work with all types of condoms. The downsides however are that they get very sticky and gooey after a little while and some women will get yeast infections or allergic reactions to the sugar-based compounds (glycerin and glycol and parabens) that make these lubes slippery. The best options for water-based lubes are the healthiest ones, like Astroglide Naturals and Good Clean Love's Almost Naked. Note that water-based lubes don't work at all in water because they just dissolve away. So, if you want super comfy sex in the hot tub or shower, you need a different kind of lube, like...

Silicone-based lubes like Eros Bodyglide, Swiss Navy and Gun Oil. These lubes have fantastic texture and staying power, and they don't get sticky like water-based lubes. However, they cannot be used with silicone dildos or any other silicone sex toy because the silicone lube bonds with the silicone toy like a glue and destroys it. Many menopausal and peri-menopausal women like the silicone lube feeling so much that they squirt a little bit inside their vaginas occasionally to give a little relief from chronic dryness. When silicone lubes eventually dry up, they just leave a silky-smooth texture like a skin moisturizer. They don't break down in water and are great for use in the shower, bath, swimming pool or ocean. They are more costly than water-based lubes, and you might have to go to a sex shop or pharmacy to find them rather than Walmart or Walgreens, but most people find they are a hundred times more enjoyable than water-based lubes and since you don't need to use as much as water-based lubes, the cost evens out in the long run.

Do not use hardware store silicone or any type of silicone other than a silicone sex lubricant! The exact silicone composition and manufacturing process is extremely important. The personal silicone sex lubricants are designed for use inside the highly absorbent and sensitive vagina, whereas the hardware store silicone lubes are built for machines and their manufacturing process leaves them with residues of chemical compounds that are toxic to the body.

Next let's talk about oils. Oils and oil-based lubes break down latex condoms, leading to reduced protection against pregnancy and STIs. Let me say that again for emphasis: oils and oil-based lubes should not be used with latex condoms although lambskin, polyurethane or nitrile condoms are fine with oil. Oils and oil-based lubes also can cause irritation, inflammation and infections such as zits in the vagina (ouch!), urinary tract infections, anal infections, candida, yeast infections and bacterial vaginosis. As such they also increase your and her risk of STI transmission, not to mention the fact that they stain sheets and are hard to clean. Overall, they are not recommended!

The one exception based on anecdotal evidence from lots of people is 100% organic cold pressed coconut oil or olive oil used in moderation. That means just use *the least amount necessary* to give enough lubrication. Don't just slobber it on! Still it is an oil, and it will clog pores and can lead to any of the health problems I just mentioned so I don't recommend it. Remember I recommend arousing her from the top down until she is so hot that she produces enough of her own lubrication, and then if you need a lubricant in addition to that then I recommend using silicone sex lube. That said, we aren't done with all the kinds of lubes. Next are…

Petroleum-based oils such as baby oil, Vaseline or mineral oil are the absolute worst you can use as they are known to contain chemicals that cause problems with regular body functions and they actually decrease your natural lubrication because they suck water out of the skin that they touch.

Vegetable oils like Crisco, soybean oil, sunflower oil and corn oil are also dangerous because the body absorbs unhealthy chemicals and components in the oils that are left over from their manufacturing processes including various industrial chemicals and highly toxic solvents that can remain in trace amounts, not to mention the trans-fats and saturated fats that are super clogging for your arteries! Just like any of the other oils I just mentioned, animal fat-based oils like butter and lard are just the same and can lead to many health problems in the vagina.

Regarding pregnancy and birth control you can get spermicidal lubricants, but they are fraught with problems and many women and men report uncomfortable or painful burning sensations after using them. The pain is due to irritation, and irritation is the breakdown of the skin. Skin that is irritated is unable to present a sealed barrier to infection and leads to increased risk of infection and STI transmission. Spermicidal lubes are not nearly as effective as a condom, and they are not nearly as comfortable as sex without a condom when the woman is really wet with arousal.

Understand that the vagina is a miraculous complex balance of pH, yeast and bacteria that are required to be in healthy balanced harmony to function properly and be delicious and smell fantastic. Industrial products made by for-profit corporations are never capable of mimicking the natural innate intelligence of the body. As such, oils and oil-based lubes, spermicidal lubricants, douches, fruits and vegetables and rubber and plastic sex toys should be used with caution and awareness that they can cause unwanted negative reactions. As a matter of respect, anything that has been used in anal sex should never be placed in the vagina unless it has been thoroughly cleaned and disinfected first! At the very least they can throw the natural balance and immunity out of homeostasis. At worst they cause bad tastes, odors, discomfort and/or full-scale infections.

You want to keep the vagina healthy and happy and properly functioning, so care for it well by learning this information and using it to protect its health for both of your pleasure and enjoyment! Women appreciate men caring for their sexual health and supporting them in their sexual care so please use the right lube for the job, which most of the time is just making sure that she is so aroused and hot that she is dripping wet and craving you before you put anything inside of her! Follow that rule and you will multiply tenfold the hotness of your sex life. Then when you need some lube assistance choose the right lube for the circumstances to support your and her sexual health and well-being. You can buy little sample packs that are about the size of a single condom to carry in your wallet or pocket and to try out different brands of lube. I highly recommend you go buy a bunch at your local adult sex shop and try them out with your partner to see what you like best and what feels best to both of your bodies. Make it fun!

Chapter 16: The Penis

Most of us received a terribly inadequate education about this extremely important organ. If it weren't for the penis and its role in reproduction none of us would be alive today! Yet most of us only learn about it from the Internet, TV shows, movies and porn… and when we use these as our sources of sex education then we inherit misconceptions, misinformation and prejudices from them. So, let's change all that, and provide you with accurate actionable intelligence about these amazing devices.

First off, over the course of a man's life he will experience many different aspects of his sexual function such as ejaculating too quickly, not being able to get hard when he wants, and being unable to have an orgasm. This is completely natural and should be embraced as part of our human experience. That said, the strength of an erection is an indicator of a man's overall health. That means that you don't have to lose erection strength when you age! If your body is fit your erection will show it. A soft or weak erection can signal emotional or mental issues like depression or anxiety, lifestyle issues like excessive stress, or physical issues like loss of tonicity of the PC muscle, cardiac issues or prostate problems. So, don't take your erections lightly! They are important!

Studies indicate that the average length of sexual intercourse is just three minutes. That's way too short for it to be very good at getting the woman off, not to mention that it's an awfully short time to spend enjoying such an amazing activity! Increasing your penis health increases your ability to last longer by increasing your stamina and staying power.

Men in top sexual health with excellent sex education and a deep relationship with their arousal and ejaculation patterns can better control their ejaculations and choose when (and if) they want to release. It's an improvement that is worthwhile for both you and your partner, as well as being a huge confidence booster.

I recommend getting control of your orgasms, but I don't recommend abstaining from ejaculation for weeks, months or years at a time. As men age they tend to experience more long-term energy reduction after ejaculating, so they naturally may not feel up to ejaculating frequently. However abstaining from ejaculation for weeks, months or years at a time (for any reason) can contribute to prostate problems. Men over 40 must deal with the very real risk of prostate hardening and prostate cancer. The prostate needs regular frequent orgasms and ejaculations to stay flexible and healthy. My view on it is "use it or lose it" because one way that we keep the prostate and penis healthy through regular sexual use. I advocate getting control over your orgasms (so that you experience the confidence boosting benefits of controlling when you ejaculate) but still choosing to ejaculate frequently (at least a once a week) to maintain a healthy functioning penis and prostate.

We'll cover how to last longer in bed in Chapter 27, and another interesting health fact is that your penis needs to have erections in order to stay healthy. It's a self-reinforcing feedback loop. The more erections you have the better your erections will be, and the less erections you have the worse they will get. Erections nourish the tissues of your penis with blood which makes the cells flexible.

Lack of blood flow dries them out and makes the cell walls more brittle and rigid. The more flexible and healthier your penis' cells are, the more blood they can fill with. Your penis will literally be able to hold more blood if it is healthy. That means it'll be bigger! So, if you want a larger penis you need to have a healthier penis. Short cuts like buying and using a cock ring (a rubber band-like ring that wraps around the penis base and neck of the scrotum like a tight bracelet) are good for helping you get and maintain a strong erection during any single sex session, but the problem is that they don't increase your penis health. They are an artificial support that doesn't assist you to become healthier and more powerful, and I advocate tools that make you stronger.

Physical fitness enthusiasts have known for years (and science has finally accepted it) that physical exercise can increase the size and health of body tissues. With regular correct exercise the penis tissues can be made more supple and stretchy, thereby resulting in a larger penis with bigger, fuller, stronger erections. The exercise to accomplish this you've hopefully already been doing since you started this book, so you should already be experiencing more frequent erections that are larger, harder and last longer! That's why

I introduced Kegels to you right away so that you could start practicing them immediately, but if you haven't started them yet then please return to Chapter 2 for the basic workout routine.

While the Kegels exercise the penis anatomy directly and locally, overall cardiovascular health and nutritional health affects it indirectly and systemically. This is because low cardiovascular fitness and bad nutrition cause low sexual stamina, underwhelming ejaculations and soft erections. Simply walking, running or exercising a few times a week and eating a majority of healthy foods will improve your penis health and sexual health by making you more energetic and fit overall.

The more fit your heart is the stronger your erections will be. Your orgasms will be more powerful because the heart is able to well irrigate the genital tissues with blood and oxygen--enhancing penile rigidity, erection time & ejaculation strength. Cardiovascular disease and heart attack have been shown to directly correlate to erectile dysfunction, but even declining cardiovascular health can impact sexual performance and satisfaction long before any actual disease or heart attack occurs. Cardiovascular health is greatly based on physical fitness and diet. Low cardiovascular health can result in things like a soft erection and an orgasm with only one or two contraction--with those contractions only seeping the ejaculate out rather than spurting it out strongly.

The good news is that increasing cardiovascular health can increase erection quality, increase orgasmic contractions (for example to as many as five to ten per orgasm), and increase the strength of the contractions enough to spray the ejaculate up to one to two feet in the air. Such things indicate to both you and your partner that you are sexually fit, youthful and vibrant!

Again, your behavior creates a feedback loop. If you are not exercising and are eating mostly unhealthy foods, then you will have decreasing sexual performance and satisfaction. That in turn leads to a low self-confidence that in turn worsens your sexual performance and satisfaction. On the flip side, if you are exercising and eating well and doing Kegels daily then you will experience a boost in self-confidence that, combined with the physical improvements, in turn further improves your sexual performance and satisfaction.

Momentum and commitment are magic. Simply start on the path and stay with it and it will self-reinforce and pick up speed over time like a snowball becoming an avalanche. You will get more and more sexually fit faster and faster simply by being consistent.

So, ask yourself, are you satisfied with the current quality of your erections, your staying power and the quality of your orgasms? Do you dribble a drop or two when you finish peeing? Do you get strong morning erections, and do they last a long time, or are they weak and short lived or nonexistent? This is extremely valuable information that you need to take note of for your own health and satisfaction in life! This is the only body you are ever going to have and if it's going downhill you are the only one who can stop it!

If you haven't been doing your Kegels, go back to Chapter 2 and start today. If you aren't exercising regularly then start doing something now. It's fine to start small like with a few pushups or a 15-minute walk, but just make sure you do it as close to every single day as you can because the effects are cumulative. Also, if you aren't eating mostly healthy fresh foods with a decent amount of fruits and vegetables and drinking at least half a gallon of water a day, then make a plan and start doing it! You will feel and be so much better for it after just a few days.

Note: It's better to start small and achieve success than to try to start big and fail. For example, it's better to say you'll do 10 pushups a day and actually succeed at doing them, than to say you'll work out an hour a day and then fail because it's too much. When I started my fitness routine all I could manage was 10 pushups a day, but I kept at it. It only took a minute to do, and I did it in the morning to get it out of the way. Over time they became easier and then I naturally wanted to start doing more. A year later and I was still doing them and had improved my health significantly. Just doing the pushups cleared up my chronic lower back pain (due to the increased core strength I gained) and gave me fuller and stronger erections (due to my increased cardiovascular fitness). So, start small and keep at it!

Now that we've covered penis health, let me tell you some penis facts.

First understand that in addition to being bad for your general health, smoking makes your penis smaller. The effect of the smoke is that it makes cell walls more rigid so they are less elastic and can't swell as much. Smoking regularly actually has been shown to decrease penis size by around ½ inch in length and ½ inch in girth. The good news is that quitting smoking and doing Kegels can recover the lost size!

While we're on the topic of penis size, most men who I've interviewed are self-conscious about the size of their penis and wish it was bigger because they feel that they would be more desirable and attractive and better in bed. I'm so humbled to have so many men be so honest with me about such a personal thing that we never talk about, and it's shown me how epidemic this shame is that most of us carry about not being as big as we wish we were. I've also interviewed hundreds of women and asked them about penis size, and the overwhelming majority say the same thing: they prefer average size men, big cocks intimidate them and that it's much better to have a lover with an average penis who understands how to use it well than to have a big cock pound her mindlessly into pain!

The adage is: "It's not the size of the boat, it's the motion in the ocean." In other words, in terms of pleasing a woman sexually, sensually and erotically, it's much more important how you touch her with your penis, body and mind than it is what size or shape your penis is.

I'll just be honest with you. I'm completely average size. I always look in the mirror and wish I was bigger, especially after seeing all the men with huge cocks in porn movies! It's completely unrealistic to compare ourselves to them both in terms of size and stamina. Those men have the biggest penises of anyone on the planet. They are representative of the very small minority of men that have penises longer than 7-inches erect length. Also, many of them are taking erectile dysfunction drugs to maintain their erections for that long. They are professionals and are not a reasonable basis for comparing average male penis size and sexual stamina! Would you use an Olympic athlete as a basis of comparison for physical health for an average person? No! It's their full-time job to maintain that level of physical fitness, and average people like you and I can't dedicate all our resources to just our physical fitness! Remember, the overwhelming majority of women enjoy average because it fits well and feels good!

No matter what size your penis is, keeping it in good health (see Chapter 2) and understanding how to use it to please a woman are the most important things. I have developed a pussy massage technique that completely redefines how to use your penis for a woman's pleasure. It is based on a deep understanding of anatomy, physiology and (of course) many hours of field testing. See the Conscious Cock Technique in the recommended resources section in Appendix A for a link to a sexually-explicit NSFW (not suitable for work) instructional video about this revolutionary technique.

We all know that a lot of men are circumcised. What many people don't know is how bad circumcision can be for men's sexual health and ability to relate deeply with women. The foreskin that is cut away removes a part of our sexual anatomy that evolved over millennia to facilitate sexual pleasure and effectiveness. The cutting away of the foreskin greatly reduces the penis' sensitivity to pleasure because it cuts and kills thousands of pleasure nerves, and intercourse is found to be less satisfying and less emotionally intimate and pleasurable for both partners because of the loss of skin's mobility over the shaft of the penis. In an uncircumcised penis the foreskin slides over the shaft liberally acting like a built-in lubricant from a position of being retracted (left in the following image) to being extended over and protecting the head (right in the following image). The effect of the foreskin is an effortless gliding motion without chafe for either partner that facilitates a sense of deeper connection and pleasure. Intercourse feels delicious and more emotionally fulfilling for both the man and the woman when the foreskin is

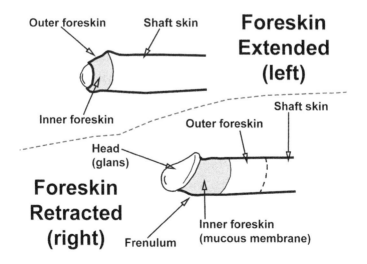

intact.

The penis is meant to function with a foreskin and biologically it isn't meant to be removed. So if you are uncircumcised then you are in the lucky minority, but if you are circumcised like most men are then know that it is actually possible to regrow your foreskin and it will help you recover lost sensitivity and the deeper connection with your partner that comes with having more skin to slide on the shaft. It's a slow process called foreskin restoration that requires tools to stretch the skin, but over time the cells multiply into new tissue. See the recommended resources section of Appendix A for links to the two big foreskin restoration forums, and if you have any questions please post them in our Facebook group.

If you are circumcised, I highly recommend that you get some good silicone sexual lubricant (like Pur, Eros Bodyglide or Swiss Navy) to help reduce chafe and soreness for you and your partner--even if you don't think it is necessary. It can make the world of difference *for her* to experience your cock as more pleasurable than the rubbing and chafing that happens between the vaginal wall and an uncircumcised penis' outer skin.

Now let's get into something fun. The part of the penis with the most pleasure receptors is called the frenulum or f-spot. It's the small area just behind the urethral opening on the underside of the penis. The ridge of the head of the cock is typically thought of as the most sensitive spot, but the frenulum is connected to two different sets of nerve bundles (the dorsal nerve and perineal nerve) while the ridge is connected to only one (the dorsal nerve).

Frenulum

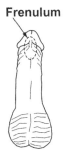

From the urethral opening back about ½ inch to one inch on the underneath of the penis is this most sensitive area, and it loves lubricated circular and back and forth flicking motions with tongues and fingers and vibrators. Many men can orgasm just from flicking motions with deep to medium pressure on this one spot alone, so feel free to share this information with your partner. Not only that but many men discover that a powerful vibrator held firmly right on this spot can make them orgasm in under a minute!

If you have any questions or if you aren't perfectly satisfied with your penis and erections and want some help but don't know where to start, then please post your thoughts, questions, experiences and comments in the Facebook group (see Appendix A). Otherwise please make an appointment with a urologist to get a checkup and some professional advice. Your Kegels, exercise and diet are the key to a healthier penis and better sex life and hopefully you're doing the Kegel exercises and are already experiencing the benefits of stronger erections and more urinary control.

Chapter 17: Semen

Whether you call it sperm, cum, ejaculate, milk, cream, jizz or something else, the proper anatomical term is semen. Sperm--the little cells with wiggly tails whose sole purpose in life is to fertilize the woman's egg to create a baby--are only about 1% to 5% of the total semen volume, so calling a man's ejaculate "sperm" is incorrect. Here we are going to shift your perspective on semen and show you that it is actually an amazing healthful substance to be revered, not some gross disgusting thing that should be avoided or felt bad about.

Semen is a potent mix of at least 50 amazing compounds. These include vitamins, minerals, enzymes, potassium, zinc, selenium, copper, calcium, magnesium, vitamin B12, amino acids, potassium, and nutritional components protein, citric acid and fructose. It's a veritable multivitamin, and it also has a powerful mix of mood elevating hormones including serotonin and oxytocin which uplift one's mood and creates feelings of love, relaxation, trust and safety.

That's an amazing list of benefits from the components that make up semen, but to benefit from them the semen needs to be absorbed into the bloodstream. A study at the University of Albany found that women who take semen into their vaginas suffer from depression less than women who use condoms. That's probably because the components of semen are easily absorbed by the vaginal wall, and even if the semen is swallowed in the mouth or received in the anus during anal sex, it is still absorbed into the bloodstream.

Note that some women may be allergic to semen however, so if your partner experiences any negative physical reaction like itching, rash or discomfort of any kind then go see a doctor. Allergic or not, if she doesn't want to take your semen inside of her then respect her preference and don't push it. If she is allergic, then it could be because your semen is too acidic because of your diet.

If she doesn't want to take your cum inside of her *don't take it personally*. It's not about you. It's about her point of view about semen. You can always circle back later and respectfully bring up the topic and explain why you want to do it, but make sure you are being honest about whether you want her to do it because you want to cum inside of her for your pleasure. Trying to sell the health benefits of it when you really just want to do it for your pleasure is a deceptive tactic that you shouldn't use. Be real and honest. Giving her accurate information about your desires and the health benefits of semen and then respecting her decision is the conscious cock way to do it. If you want to share the health benefits with her then watch the "Vitamin BJ" video by Kim Anami together with her, and then ask what she thinks, and then follow her lead. The video link is in the recommended resources section in Appendix A in the back of this book.

Many women who are deeply in love with a man may report craving their partner's semen--literally feeling a need to receive it, be filled with it, taste it or rub it over their skin. Many other women don't like the taste or smell of semen, however. I suspect that's because many men have bad diets that make their semen taste horrible. I firmly believe that you should know how you taste. If you want your partner to like your semen and, for example, to want you to come in her mouth, then I think it's only ethical that you know what you taste like and try to make your semen taste as good as possible. Cut down on coffee, alcohol and cigarettes, eat less red meat and dairy products, drink lots of water to stay hydrated (aim for a gallon a day), and specifically eat more celery, citrus and lots of naturally sweet fruits like pineapple, apples, melons, grapes, mangos, bananas and strawberries. A man who has such a good diet usually has sweet and savory tasting semen rather than sour and bitter. You can taste it yourself to see. Just dip your finger in it and dab a tiny bit on the tip of your tongue. You don't have to swallow, and you don't have to taste any more than a dab. It's a great way to easily check your overall dietary health.

Next let's move on to STI transmission through semen. Condoms are a necessary and important protection against sexually transmitted infections and pregnancy. However, if both you and your partner are interested in having intercourse without condoms and both of you want you to ejaculate inside her, then I recommend doing the following. First, go get tested for STIs together with your partner, and find out your current STI-statuses. Then pick & choose a different form of birth control together and start using it rather than condoms. There's nothing better than a juicy sexfest when you are both completely relaxed because you have no fear of infections or pregnancy, but you must be conscious about the decision *beforehand* in order to access this paradise.

Semen can contain any STI that is transmitted by body fluids, but if you don't have any of those infections then your semen is STI-free. And if you get a vasectomy then your semen is sperm-free. If your semen is both STI-free and sperm-free then you can't get your partner pregnant and you can't give her an STI... and if you eat a good diet and your semen tastes good then your semen can be a joyous and even delightful substance for both of you, rather than something threatening, scary or yucky. It completely changes the rules of the game and redefines semen from something threatening to something yummy!

Now for a couple of side notes. First, facials are all the rage today in porn. If you don't know, a facial is where a man ejaculates on a woman's face. Some women like facials and some women hate them. Some find it luscious and some find it demeaning. So make sure you check in with her about the idea *before trying it*, and understand that if the semen gets in her eye it will hurt and burn a lot. Also, realize that if you have any STIs you can transmit them to her if your semen comes into contact with her eye or the inside her nose or mouth. So, if you want to come on her face then make sure that you are STI-free *first,* and then ask her if she would like you to do it to her, and if so, how would she like it? Perhaps she'd rather that you cum on her belly and that she rubs it onto her face with her fingers, for instance. If she doesn't want to do it then just drop the idea respectfully and replace it with something that is empowering to her that she likes instead.

Second, I can't say it enough that you really need to protect against pregnancy. It was recently found that semen also contains a hormone called ovulation-inducing factor which signals the female to release hormones that trigger ovulation which means that regardless of where she is in her menstrual cycle, *the mere presence of semen in her vagina can trigger ovulation*! This explains why so many women get pregnant when practicing the rhythm method of birth control, so there's no fooling around here. Be conscious and use this knowledge to wield the power of sex to fuel your relationship and infuse it with amazing energy while simultaneously respecting its power to create life! Remember that all bodily fluids--including semen--can carry STIs, so be sure to get tested and have your partner tested before playing with the magical mystical powers of semen.

Chapter 18: Nipples

Nipples and breasts are a powerful erogenous zone for women, but you must know how to touch them properly. Men often don't know what to do with them and end up being clumsy and ineffective, too rough and just grabbing and squeezing them or avoiding them entirely because they aren't sure how to handle them. Let's solve that mystery once and for all and empower you to understand them and unlock their sex super powers!

Touch that is too fast, too rough, too intense or too anything can be annoying or even painful. The key here is to understand subtlety and intensity. Many women have never had a man be an attentive lover so as to learn to enjoy nipple play. So be aware, she might not think it'll be enjoyable to begin with.

First, let's talk about anatomy and the neural-mechanics of the nipples. Scientific research at Rutgers University published in the *Journal of Sexual Medicine* revealed that the nipples stimulate the exact same sensory areas of the brain that the clitoris, cervix and vagina stimulate. Nipple play also releases the exact same hormone that clitoral play releases: oxytocin, which assists sexual arousal, triggers uterine contractions, decreases anxiety and depression, and increases bonding and trust! You can get all of that just from nipple play without even getting into her pants. Why wouldn't you want to master this art?

First you need to learn how your partner's nipples look when she's not aroused and how they look when she's fully turned on--like after she's had an orgasm. Notice the difference in size, height, width, texture, fullness and density. By learning how her nipples are when she's aroused and when she's completely not aroused you will be able to use them as an indicator of her level of arousal. For her it's extremely easy. She can see if your cock is erect, but for you to look at her and read her level of arousal is a finer art. Learning to wield the tool of nipple-reading will help you to become a more masterful lover.

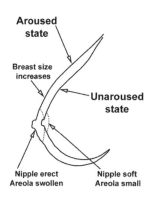

Aroused state

Breast size increases

Unaroused state

Nipple erect Areola swollen — **Nipple soft Areola small**

In general, a woman's non-aroused nipples are very soft, smaller and less raised, and the areola (the pink part around the nipple that is part of the nipple and not part of the breast) is not swollen. When they get aroused the nipples perk up like a little penis and the areola engorges and swells. The nipple gets harder and firmer and more sensitive... just like your erect cock when you are turned on. This is because they are both composed of erectile tissue that responds to arousal levels by getting erect!

The basic method of playing with a woman's nipples that I recommend is to start slow and light and tease with occasional touch with the very tip of your tongue because it is so sensitive and subtle. It's also great to use your fingers, but you must be extremely aware and conscious because you can easily be too rough and lose the window of opportunity by *overwhelming her sensitivity* and putting her into sensory overload where your touch does nothing for her. With super light fingertip touching and tracing and an occasional light squeeze quickly followed by a slight flicking of the nipple, you can cause a delicious shockwave of sensation to ripple through the body. Try it on yourself first to develop your sensitivity and skill because you have the same nervous system pathways and nipple sensitivity as a woman. This is something that you must do carefully and not too much at the beginning, but when mastered, often this pulse of energy can travel directly to her clitoris and make it throb with surges of pleasure from just your careful teasing of her nipples while staying very in-tune with her reactions and experience.

As she warms up more and more, then your nipple touch can probably get more frequent with heavier pressure. But don't rush it and don't overdo it! Check in with her and stay tuned to her signals. Let them guide you! It may be totally true that when she's really warmed up you can squeeze and flick them harder and even constantly. However, the opposite technique of teasing them with only an occasional flick or squeeze and then long time-spans without touching them may provide more intense shockwaves for her. She will be your teacher if you pay attention to her signals.

However, if you can't tell what she likes and what she doesn't like by reading her body language then ask her what type of nipple touch she likes and doesn't like *right now* (as in--at this moment. See Appendix E). It can change in a minute so don't assume it'll be guaranteed to work next time. With attention you may be able to determine that she has a general nipple stimulation pattern, but any single moment or single sexual encounter may be different so stay in touch with what's happening *each time*.

For example, you might learn that during initial contact before any arousal has yet taken place that she likes long, slow, wispy tracing strokes of your fingers on her breast and around her nipple - with only a very occasional single quick light flick and that when she is a bit further along in early arousal, she likes you to squeeze them gently for a second and then release gently with no flick, and then later when she's completely aroused and hot she wants you to have both nipples in a deep squeeze with regular flick-offs that help her to orgasm while grinding on your cock.

She also might be so sensitive that she experiences sensory overload like you probably do right after you orgasm--when you can't have the head of your cock stimulated for a minute! You don't want to burst a bliss-bubble so read her body language and check in with her frequently.

Remain mindful and present and don't get so carried away that you lose your sensitivity to her signals--like the sounds she makes, how she's breathing and the way she opens or closes her body to you. Don't get carried away and become a vise grip on her nipple or twist it until it hurts. She won't appreciate that, and your lack of sensitivity will not engender her to trust you with her sensitive nipples.

It's an amazing sex super power when you master the art of playing with her nipples. Many women have found that when they are in a high state of arousal, like for example after they have already had an orgasm or two, properly timed and executed nipple play can trigger another orgasm for them because nerves from the nipples can trigger clitoral, vaginal and uterine contractions! What an amazing magical power to explore!

Remember every woman is different, and every woman herself is different at any moment depending on all the factors going on in her life and her heart and brain. To empower the mutual pleasure of the experience, communicate with her, read her subtle cues and ask her directly with your words when you aren't sure or aren't getting clear or congruent body language messages. Track her well, and she will love you for the dedication you give her and will respond by being more trusting and willing to open and be your sex partner and Goddess.

Chapter 19: The Clitoris

The clitoris is an amazing device. Its only function is sexual pleasure, and it has about 8,000 nerve endings, which is double what a penis has! Can you imagine if your cock was twice as sensitive as it is now? Wow!

Developmentally, the clitoris is the female equivalent of the penis. During prenatal development, all of us start off with the same thing down there, called the "genital tubercle," which means bump, which develops into the "phallus" and then differentiates into either the clitoris for women or the penis for men. As such, they have many similarities like a "glans" or head, a foreskin, and a shaft, and they both are composed of erectile tissue and swell when aroused.

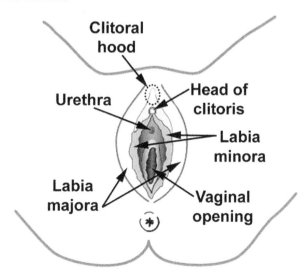

The clitoral head (as shown on previous page) is what most people know about when they think about a clitoris, but recent advances in sexual anatomy research have revealed that the clitoris actually has a very large and intricate shape inside the woman's body (as shown below), looking somewhat like a wishbone with one bulb and one leg (the corpus cavernosum) on each side of the vagina. The head is a bit in front of the urethra and vagina, and its distance away from the vaginal opening can determine whether the clitoral head gets stimulated during penis intercourse.

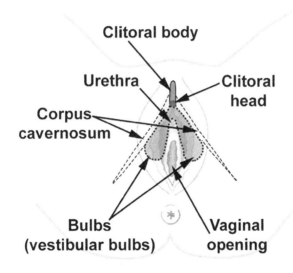

If it's far away, then the penis may completely miss the clitoris during penetration, while women with a clitoris closer to the vaginal opening may experience clitoral stimulation from penetrative sex. To improve your chances of stimulating the clitoral head during intercourse, the man can inch up until his shoulders are higher than the woman's to change the angle of entry so that his shaft can rub the nub while he thrusts.

That said, you have to understand how the clitoris works. The whole structure is composed of erectile tissue and if it isn't aroused and filled with blood then it generally doesn't feel good to be touched directly or sharply or heavily. As a woman becomes aroused and the clitoris becomes more erect, then the entire extended structure including the bulbs and corpus cavernosum become more pleasurable. This explains why when a woman is not aroused it can be annoying for her to have her clitoral head touched directly, but when she is fully aroused, she may enjoy having it stroked directly repeatedly with firm pressure and high intensity.

But just focusing on the head is a mistake. The two legs or bulbs on each side of the vagina are part of the "clit" too, and they swell up and also get sensitive. The opening of a woman's vagina is where the most nerve endings are, and inside there aren't many at all. That's because the bulbs of the clitoris surround the opening. So, you can stimulate the clit through her vaginal walls right inside the opening on the left and right sides once she is moderately to fully aroused. Think circular motions and side to side strokes.

There is a definite limit to how much stimulation feels good for the clitoris, and often when approaching climax or after climaxing it can become so sensitive that the woman no longer wants it to be touched at all. You've got to read her cues, her body language and the sounds she makes, and back off when she indicates that it's too much. When the clit becomes too sensitive to stimulate directly then it's time to turn to surrounding areas and other things, like the G-spot, penetration, caresses or kisses.

It's been reported that more than half of women need to have their clitoris stimulated in order to orgasm. Another way to say this is that intercourse alone is not sufficiently stimulating for most women to climax! By learning her sexual anatomy and varying your intercourse angle and position men can learn how to find the sweet spot and give her some delicious friction on the clitoral head during intercourse. Of course, you can always use your hands and fingers to love up the clit during intercourse to make sure that it is touched (see Chapter 27: Hand Jobs). Make sure your hands are clean, so you don't give her a urinary tract infection, and that your nails are trimmed short and filed smooth, so you don't cut her. Also, you can kiss and lick her clitoris (see Chapter 29: Oral Sex / Cunnilingus). Either way, be aware of her responses and vary your touch movement pattern, pressure and friction until you find what she likes and then keep doing that until she comes, or her cues indicate to you that she wants something different or wants to stop. There is no need to make her orgasm every time. It's perfectly enjoyable for her to just luxuriate in the pleasure without getting to orgasm.

The word "clitoris" comes from the Greek word for

"key," which shows that the Greeks knew its important role in producing pleasure for women. Learning its anatomy and how to touch and play and love it will unlock some of the mysteries of your lover's delicious orgasms, and you'll both enjoy the ride.

Chapter 20: The G-Spot

Now for the infamous G-spot. Sit back and put your learning cap on and get ready for this download because knowing more about this special place on a woman's body is going to immediately make you a better lover. First off, the G-spot is real. It absolutely exists, but it's been misunderstood for a long time. Recent research in female sexual anatomy has corrected the errors and revealed the reality of how this amazing sexual structure functions.

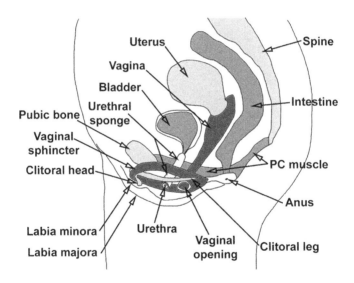

First off, it's not a spot. It's actually a sleeve around the urethra. The urethra is the tube through which pee passes from the woman's bladder when she's urinating. It's a few inches long and is just in front of the vagina (see "urethral sponge" in image above). You can think of the vagina as a large tube and the urethra as a small tube, and they generally are parallel to each other with the urethra in front of the vagina. This means that the urethra is between the woman's vagina and her belly button on her front side. The G-spot is a sleeve of spongy erectile tissue around the urethral tube, much like a man's penis is a sleeve of erectile tissue surrounding his urethral tube. And just like a penis, the G-spot expands and hardens when aroused. So now that you understand the anatomy, you can understand that the correct name for this area is the urethral sponge, not the G-spot.

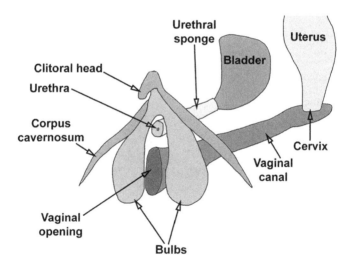

As she gets aroused, the urethral sponge (see above) fills with blood and becomes more prominent. When it becomes engorged, it also becomes much more sensitive.

The image on the next page shows how many women find stimulation of it through the front wall of the vagina (two fingers inserted and pressing against the pubic bone) to be wonderfully pleasurable. Not only that, but the clitoral shaft, legs and bulbs are all connected to it by ligaments so stimulating the urethral sponge also stimulates the clitoris, but from the inside front of the vagina!

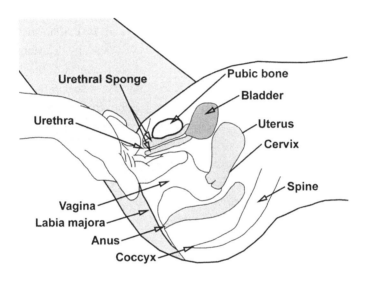

The urethral sponge contains a network of glands and ducts that are called the Skene's glands, and as the urethral sponge becomes aroused these glands fill with a sexual fluid that is now known as female ejaculate. Ten years ago, almost no one knew about female ejaculation, but nowadays the information is spreading like wildfire. If a woman's urethral sponge is stimulated sufficiently and in the right way for her, when she orgasms the contraction can send this fluid squirting out of her urethra just like a man squirts semen out of his cock when he has an orgasm. Some people call it squirting, but the correct term is female ejaculation because while some women squirt when ejaculating, others seep, others gush, and others may dribble.

It can be very disconcerting or even embarrassing for the woman if she doesn't know what is happening because it feels like she is peeing because fluid is exiting her urethra. Knowledge is power however, and by learning about what the body is doing we can alleviate these concerns by explaining that it is a natural sexual process that is producing a sexual fluid, not urine. In India female ejaculate is called "amrita" which roughly translates to "nectar of the goddess" or "water of life" and it is a sacred thing to be revered and considered holy. Consider dipping your fingers in it and anointing your third eye or heart with it as a sign of reverence and appreciation if you ever help her ejaculate.

So now that you know about it, you probably want to know how to access it and how to touch it. First off, get your head on straight. Do not even think about entering the inner sanctum of her vagina until she is very highly aroused and make sure that your hands are clean, and you have short nails that are filed smooth. Bring patience and loving attention to her and let her heat up until her vagina almost literally sucks your finger in--hungry to be filled. If you are at all unsure then ask her! Only with her permission should you ever enter, and the only way she will relax enough to have a G-spot orgasm with you is if she trusts your presence with her. When you do enter her, enter first with only one finger, slowly, consciously and carefully. Don't just jam it in. Savor the sensations on your finger and allow her to savor the sensation of being entered by a conscious lover.

For initial exploration, I recommend that she lay on a bed on her back and you enter with your palm facing to the ceiling so that you can make a "come here" motion with your finger. Take your time, explore, and play with all the erectile tissues that are just inside the entrance. As she warms up further and her vagina relaxes then slide a second finger inside so that you are using your pointer finger and middle finger side-by-side. Then curl your fingertips up towards her belly button and gently and lovingly explore for a firm spot. Try gentle back and forth motions and small circles and gently pushing up and back down and ask her what feels good. When you find the spot then explore it between your two fingers gently and slide up towards her head along it. You will find that it is a shaft that you can stroke up and down, towards her head and back down towards her feet. You can probably feel 1 to 3 inches of the engorged urethral shaft through the front wall of her vagina with your two fingertips.

Being gentle and slow at the beginning, paying attention to her cues and asking her verbally for feedback, is the way to proceed. I highly recommend playing with her clitoral head with your other hand or giving her oral sex on her clitoris while you do this. If things go well and she heats up, you may find that faster or firmer strokes on the G-spot will help her to orgasm. But she is your guide, not me, and every woman is different so ask her and let her be your teacher (See Appendix E). Do not get fixated on the goal of making her ejaculate! That will hinder your success. Instead stay focused on giving her the most pleasure *in every single moment*. There is no need for her to have an orgasm, and the only way to really get there is by following the pleasure. Otherwise if you make the orgasm your goal you can easily end up being too rough, too fast, too aggressive and tiring out your hand, not to mention overloading your partner.

The G-spot is an amazing pleasure point and any conscious lover must master how to love and adore it. If you have any questions or comments or have any successes or failures to share, please post them in the Facebook group.

Chapter 21:
The A-Spot and Cervical Orgasms

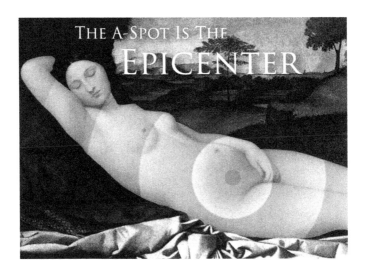

In this chapter, we are going to go deep and talk about the most profound type of orgasm that many women can ever have: a cervical orgasm. Most men have no idea how to love the cervix, and most women never get to experience the profound and all-encompassing pleasure that comes from cervical orgasms. So, open your mind if you aren't already a master of the A-spot and cervical orgasms and get ready to sexercise your brain.

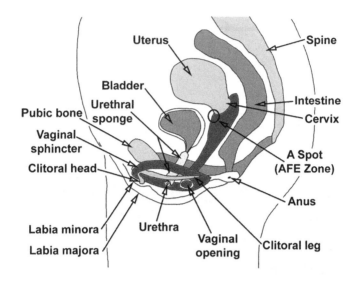

The A-spot is a little-known place inside a woman right in front of her cervix that works with the cervix to do amazing yummy things. It's also called the Anterior Fornix Erogenous zone, or the AFE zone (see above), and is also known as the epicenter. The cervix is the equivalent sexual structure to the male prostate. The A-spot is located just behind and above the G-spot just below and in front of the cervix in the innermost point of the vagina. Even though the A-spot and cervix are at the farthest end of the vagina, you don't need to have a long penis to access it. Since the vaginal canal averages around three inches long even a long finger can reach it. The cervix is shaped like a tiny doughnut (see image on the next page) and is distinctly firmer than any of the surrounding vagina. It protrudes into the vagina and can be found easily once you know where it is.

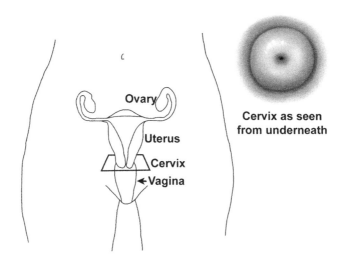

Cervix as seen from underneath

The A-spot's sexual super power is that it can produce rapid lubrication even if the woman is not very aroused yet, and the more often it is used the more effective it becomes. For some women who experience a lack of lubrication, massaging this area regularly or occasionally may alleviate chronic vaginal dryness.

Since the A-spot is right on the front side of the cervix and closely linked to it, it is one of the deepest most intimate places of a woman's body. For loving this epicenter inside of her she must be really open to you, and you must have a good emotional connection. Even if you are in a long-term relationship her heart might be closed to you and therefore, she won't be able to let you access her A-spot and her cervix. They simply will be too disturbing or scary for her and too sensitive to be touched or accessed. If this is the case, then you need to do emotional clearing and healing work to reconnect your hearts and make sure that you are deeply aligned with each other before even thinking about trying to get to know her A-spot or cervix. If you have questions about this, please post them in the Facebook group.

The benefits of learning about her A-spot and cervix are numerous and amazing. Women describe these orgasms as producing waves of pleasure through a spiritual whole-body experience when they experience a feeling of deep connection, openness, vulnerability and often may cry tears of release and joy. They can clear out sexual trauma and stuck energy and have been described as feeling like you've taken ecstasy and are experiencing spiritual enlightenment!

So, if you want to successfully venture down this juicy path of exploration you will need to understand a few things. First you are going to have to clear the air, make sure that you are emotionally connected and that she is open to you and to trying this with you. If not, then don't try it yet. But if you are both ready then you need to get in a comfortable position to try to access the A-spot and the cervix. I recommend missionary position: with her laying on her back, relaxed and with her legs open while you kneel between her legs.

For beginners I'd recommend that you don't even try to touch the A-spot or cervix until she's maybe 75% of the way to having an orgasm or has already had one or two. Then, with her well warmed up and sexually open and excited, slowly enter farther to find and explore the epicenter. You may need to massage the cervix and A-spot for 30 to 45 minutes for her to reach the orgasm, so you have to have your mind in the right place of attention and focus. You may need to shift your body's position and switch fingers or hands occasionally. Don't hurt yourself by staying in a bad position with too much tension in your hand or arm!

You have to be able to hold her "in the middle of the fire" for as long as it takes without dropping her or shrinking back. You don't want to leave her unsatisfied, or worse ungrounded and spiritually broken open, triggered and vulnerable. You must be able to stand the test of time and endurance that it takes. These orgasms are often not quick.

When or if intense emotions come up the key is to breathe deeply together with lots of eye contact and love and keep breathing through them as they come. There is absolutely no way to force this orgasm. You must open the space, hold it open and let her come to it on her own schedule. Her orgasm isn't about your manhood. Your manhood is about creating the space. Do not make the orgasm the goal. Make touching her lovingly there and sharing the delicious deep experience together the goal. You can always start small just by making contact and then at some later date in the future massage it for longer... building up over time until maybe one day you both can do it for half an hour or more.

The way to begin touching is with gentle light to

medium pressured touch in slow gentle strokes. Think gentle loving slow massage not flicking, tapping or poking. While she may enjoy having it touched gently by a dexterous and sensitive finger, having it banged into or poked repeatedly by a fucking finger or penetrating cock is going to be uncomfortable or hurt her. Men just imagine getting kicked in the balls repeatedly. That should make you feel some empathy for how intense it can be for her.

So, use some lube and gently explore with light to medium pressure in sideways strokes. It responds to pressure and movement not static touch. Experiment with a "come hither" motion of your finger, pulling gently along the front of the vagina, gentle circular motions around the cervix (remember it is shaped like a small circular doughnut), gliding over it until she experiences total body pleasure. Remember: gentle pressure and slow continuous motion, not poking!

Around ovulation the cervix is very high up and tends to be more likely to produce cervical orgasms. During menstruation the cervix lowers and is more likely to feel pain and discomfort when touched. Cervical orgasms produce more oxytocin than clitoral orgasms, and unlike the clitoris which feels too sensitive to be touched for a while after an orgasm, the cervix has no refractory period and can continue to be stroked and stimulated non-stop, leading to ongoing rolling never-ending orgasm possibilities!

The best position for many people for success at A-spot and cervical orgasms from penile vaginal intercourse is with the man on his back laying down and the woman on top straddling him. There she can take him inside and then wiggle up a little bit towards his head or down towards his feet to get the angle of penetration right so that the head of his cock rests on the A-spot or cervix. Then she can gyrate her hips to produce a side-to-side massaging motion or grind front-to-back. Both are better for cervical and A-spot stimulation than an in-and-out motion. Many women report quick delicious lubrication appearing this way as she can control the depth, pressure, rhythm and intensity and get it right...on...the...*perfect*...spot, in a way that a man never could since it's not in his body.

Section 4:

Stoke the Fire: Intimacy Tools

Chapter 22: Eliminating Negativity

Next, we are going to cover another one of the most important things that you can do to improve your relationship: removing all negativity from it. Basically, negativity is any thought, word or action that communicates to your partner that she is not okay when she thinks or acts the way that she does. There are the obvious forms of negativity like insults, shaming and criticizing, but there are also many subtler forms like so called constructive criticism, putdowns, dismissals, inattention, sounding bored, flippant hurtful judgments, and rolling your eyes. Whatever it is, the message is that one person is superior, and the other person is inferior.

All aspects of negativity poison any potential safe-space that you have in your relationship and are toxic to the process of true connection and love. At its core, negativity is a form of abuse and you can look at it like a toxicity that is poisoning a natural water supply. If you remove the toxicity, then eventually the water supply will become clean and potable again. You don't want to repress your feelings towards your partner, but rather to look at them with a critical eye and recognize them as signs that something about your relationship needs attention. It's a two-way street, so this technique is best employed by both of you working together rather than you doing it alone.

The things about your partner that bring out your negativity really are your responsibility. She is just being herself, but you get angry because she's not being *the way that you want her to be*. She's failing to meet your unspoken needs. No one is responsible for meeting your unspoken needs except you! That is how children act. They expect their parents to meet their unspoken needs because that's what parents do! But when we grow up and mature into adulthood it's not healthy to transfer that expectation onto our partners. She isn't your mother and therefore shouldn't be expected to meet your unspoken needs.

Honestly, the best way to solve problems in your relationship is to see how you are contributing to them! The rewards of doing this are immense. By eliminating all negativity in your relationship, you will begin to automatically focus on your partner's good points, just like you did when you were new lovers together. You'll start seeing things in a more positive way. You'll see her as she *really is* rather than scolding her for not fitting the image you have in your mind of who you *want her to be*. Examples of negativity include criticizing her, stonewalling her, invading her space, avoiding her, shaming her, correcting her, gaslighting her, showing her contempt, making fun of her and insulting her. Many people use these techniques both consciously and unconsciously to try to bully their partner into compliance.

It can be grossly disgusting when you really understand it for what it is--two people beating each other up to try to force the other to meet their unspoken needs. The negativity that you throw at your partner just comes back to bite you in the ass anyway. The stress hormone cortisol (that a person produces when being physically attacked) is also produced in the person doing the attacking. You end up being biochemically, physically and emotionally trashed if you attack her with negativity, and she, of course, feels trashed because you beat her up. It's a form of self-abuse *and* partner abuse when you realize this.

So, get rid of that sick tactic. Eliminate all negativity in your relationship and start seeing, loving and appreciating your partner for who she really is and what she does to help your relationship. It will help you to create a safe-space in which a healthy sex life and love life can grow. A great tactic to choose to implement is that for every negative comment that happens counteract it with three positive comments. For me, I recommend simply quitting cold-turkey. Enough of the bullshit already. Stop taking out your frustration at your unmet needs on her and start *meeting your own needs* while fostering a safe-space free of all forms of negativity. I guarantee you it will help you, your partner, your relationship and your sex life.

But how do you actually do it? How do you stop being negative? We often don't know we're being negative. We cloud our judgment about how we really are acting, often thinking we're being helpful and constructive while in reality we are being hurtful and negative. All our ideas about how our partner can improve herself and do things better can be negative, correcting, nagging behaviors. Correcting with love is for parents not for partners. Removing negativity doesn't mean that you don't get frustrated anymore, but rather it means that you find a different and positive way to express that frustration. Again, for best results *you both* should do it, but even if you just do it by yourself you will experience significant improvement in the quality of your relationship.

1. You must admit when your partner has hurt you. That takes courage because it's the person who gets hurt who must tell the one who did the hurting! However, compared to getting hurt repeatedly until you leave (or feel like leaving), telling her is comparatively much easier. Here you are training your partner about what you consider to be a put-down, dismissal or negative judgment.

2. When your partner puts you down (either intentionally or by accident, or in a new way), you must control your reaction because you aren't allowed to feed the fire by saying a negative "tit for tat" defensive comeback. Instead of repeating a put-down/comeback cycle, you must *choose to respond* in a way that breaks the cycle. For example, you can say, "I bet that what you just said is important to you, and I want to understand it, but all I hear is a put-down (or insult or dismissal, etc.) even if you didn't mean it that way. Can you please say that in a different way that isn't negative to me?" This shines the light on what they just did and gives them an opportunity to try it again. In this way you support yourself *and* you support your partner by improving their communication technique. By extension, if you catch yourself slipping and being negative or putting your partner down in some way you can stop yourself and apologize, and then try again and say it in a positive way. For example, instead of saying, "These laundry sheets you buy smell like crap,"

you could say, "I don't like how these laundry sheets smell. Can we pick out a different kind that we both like sometime?"

3. Counteract the negativity with some positivity! Each night when you go to bed give each other positive encouragement and appreciation. To do this both of you simply share with each other three things that you saw the other person do that made your lives better that day. Keep at it every night, even when it's hard and even when you can't come up with anything. Expressing appreciation and gratitude is a powerful way to keep up leveling your experience of a happy and fulfilled life and to attract more of what you really want into your relationship.

4. Keep track so that it gets easier over time! Put a calendar of the month on the wall in the kitchen or bathroom to help you stay accountable and track your progress. When you both get through a 24-hour day without saying anything negative to each other put a gold star or smiley face sticker on the calendar. To do this you both have to work together as a team to achieve the sticker. You can hold each other accountable to not let each other down, and it can be a powerful motivator that bonds you together. Keep at it until you can get through a whole month without either of you even once being negative to the other.

This technique is about retraining your brain to not keep doing the negative communication patterns that you used to think were normal baseline behavior. It has saved many relationships, so don't underestimate its power. Go get some gold stars and a calendar and start it today.

Chapter 23: Rekindling the Fire

Let's get into rekindling the fire in your relationship. Tell your partner that you want to do a little exercise with her to get to know her better because you love her, and you want to learn to love her better. Then when you have some quiet time alone get a couple pieces of paper and pens and sit down and ask her to write a list of ten things that if you were to do them, they would make her feel loved by you. At the same time, you write down on your paper ten things that, if your partner did them, they would make you feel loved by her.

Let's investigate that just a little bit to help you understand the exercise better. The basic idea is that by sharing with each other specific information about what pleases you, and by agreeing to do things on a regular basis that please your partner, you start to take full ownership of what your needs and desires are and create a safe-space between you. Now, notice that I said, "if you were to do them." None of these are required. After you both finish your lists, then exchange them. Next pick a couple or a few of the things on the list that are *easy for you to do* and start doing them for your partner lovingly, freely and regularly. You can't do them begrudgingly, nor with any expectation of something in return. They have to be freely given in order to be received as acts of love!

Now, let's recognize that it can be scary to share what we really, really want with our partners. So, let me encourage you, if you are feeling scared, to start small with simple easy things. Just make sure that they are real. You can always test the waters with little things and then go deeper in the future if this works out well. Be kind with yourself and with her.

Out of the ten things that she listed that if you did them, she would feel loved, some will surely not be things that you are willing or want to do. That's fine and to be expected! However, there will surely be a few things that you can easily say, "Yes, absolutely I can do that for you!" That's what you are looking for, the items that you can do with excitement and joy! Do them, do them regularly and do them with grace and pleasure *with no expectation of anything in return.*

Now that you understand the exercise let's look at some examples to get your mental juices rolling. You can start off by beginning sentences in your mind with: "I feel loved when you…" If you recall something that she used to do, but doesn't do any more you could say, "I used to feel loved when you…" If it's something that she's never done, you could say, "I would feel loved if you…"

They can be anything, like for example:

- Massage me for an hour
- Tell me that you love me every day
- Shower with me
- Try the 69-sex position
- Surprise me with a present
- Cook me a special meal

134

- Go on a date with me once a month
- Make love X times a day/week/month
- Open the door for me
- Make a sexy video together
- Read a novel to me at bedtime
- Compliment how I look
- Kiss me when you leave

You see, they must be real world tangible things in order to count. "Treat me better" or "love me more" aren't concrete enough to work here. You must have measurable things for this to work.

When your partner does any of the things that you would like her to do to make you feel loved, you absolutely must acknowledge it with verbal appreciation. Say thank you! Tell her it makes you feel wonderful when she does that for you. And when you do these things for your partner, make sure that you do them no matter how you are currently feeling about her. If you are mad at her or annoyed by her, do them anyway! That's when they matter and count the most, and it shows that you are committed and congruent, and that she can count on you! Do these even if you feel resistance, and after a while they'll get easier and come naturally to you. And if you are in a new or young relationship, understand that doing these things helps you set a solid foundation for long-term success.

Chapter 24: True Listening

Most people aren't taught how to really listen. They actually filter and distort what other people say with their own thoughts and perceptions, and I guarantee you that if you don't master the art of listening there are going to be times when you miss chances for deep juicy connection with your partner. It's not hard to do, but you must know how and luckily there's only three simple steps:

Step #1: Mirror what she says. This step can be hard to do. When she says something important, repeat it back to her as closely as you can and ask if you got it right. What you are trying to do here is demonstrate that you heard and understood her *exactly*, without putting any words in her mouth or distorting the meaning that she was trying to convey. After you say it back to her then ask her, is that what you meant? Did I get it right? If she says no then listen to her clarify it, and then repeat that back to her until she says that you got it right. It's a sure-fire way to make sure that you really understand each other and aren't interpreting what she's saying through your mental lens rather than hearing what she's trying to communicate from her perspective. It might feel like "parroting," but I encourage you to trust the process as every step builds to something greater.

Sometimes however just hearing accurately isn't enough for true listening. Sometimes you must go even farther. That leads us to Step #2: Validation. Here the goal is to understand your partner's point of view. You don't have to agree with it now, but you must demonstrate that you can see her perspective and that you can see that it makes sense to her from her perspective. You basically are demonstrating that you: a) are mature enough to see something from someone else's point of view even if you disagree, and b) that you can reassure her that she isn't crazy just for having a different opinion than you!

I think most men get lots of mileage out of always making their partner feel like she is wrong, illogical or crazy, and it boosts his ego while demeaning her. If you want a better relationship, then learn to validate her point of view by seeing her perspective after accurately listening to what she explains. Then imagine it from her perspective. Imagine you were her. Then (if you can imagine it the way she sees it) tell her that you can see her opinion from her point of view and that you can see how it makes sense to her. It doesn't mean that you must agree or approve. It just means that you acknowledge the sanity, truth and validity of her opinions and perception.

Some things require even deeper skills than validating, and here we come to Step #3: Empathy. This can be hard for a lot of guys who live in their thinking rational minds all the time because it requires that you shift your focus into your feeling sensory awareness. Basically, to empathize you must put yourself in her shoes and imagine how she feels after: a) understanding what she said and, b) realizing that her opinion makes sense from her point of view.

Empathizing gives you the experience of what your partner is feeling as if it were happening to you. Let's say that it's really important to her that you get her a card for her birthday, but you forget. In order to empathize with her experience you have to imagine how she feels, *not how you think that she should feel*. The sensations and emotions become clear to you when you feel it in your body and heart as if you were actually her. It requires volitional conscious imagination if you aren't used to doing it. When you can feel the pain that she is sharing and sit in the middle of it with her and demonstrate that you "get it" ...that is truly powerful healing and connection. The idea is to let go of all your judgments and opinions and try to imagine and experience *how it feels to her.*

None of this is a one-way street. The best is when you both can do these three steps with each other whenever they are needed. It will bring you much closer together and can heal wounds and turn them into fertilizer to help your relationship grow even stronger and sexier than ever before.

When both of you mirror, validate and empathize with each other, you defuse landmines and can love each other because you understand each other and demonstrate your interest in connecting to each other more than in being right. It shows her that you really *get her world* without invalidating your perspective. That's powerful relationship medicine. Just remember that making changes like this don't happen all at once. We are human so be sure to cut yourself some slack because we rarely can do everything perfectly, especially the first few times. It helps to be flexible, forgiving and kind to yourself and to your partner. Give these techniques time and practice and they will reveal layer after layer of gifts to you.

Chapter 25:
How to Ask for What You Really Want

It's often difficult to ask for what we really want. We can be afraid of judgment or backlash. We can fear that asking will reveal a part of ourselves that we have kept hidden. We may think our desire is shameful or bad. We may simply not know how or when to bring it up--never finding the right words or the right moment. We may think that it's impossible and just resign ourselves to complacency. All these things result in paralysis.

When we don't ask for what we really want, we are inauthentic. It causes us to play a role and act as if we are someone we are not. So many people live their entire lives in a prison where they never ask for what they really want, and this inauthenticity can lead to depression, anxiety, a feeling of hopelessness, anger or despair. Many turn to alcohol or other types of addiction, and all of this can be avoided by learning how to ask for what we really want!

Asking doesn't mean you'll get it, but it does mean that you'll have a chance to! You'll miss 100% of the shots you never make. You must take a chance to have a chance.

But how do we do it when we are afraid that our desire is going to cause problems in our relationship? How do we find the right time and place? How do we find the right words? I don't know anyone who learned this stuff in school, and it is one of the most important skills we can have to live a fulfilled life, for if we can't advocate for ourselves no one else is going to do it for us.

To start with, you have to get your perspective right. Realize that *you may have been thinking a lot about the thing you want to ask for but for your partner it might be a completely new idea.* She may need time to think about it and adjust to it. You must expect that she will need an acceptance and acculturation period. Be ready to sit through it as it takes its course. It will not proceed on your timeline. It will proceed on hers. You need to be able to accept that and work with it at her speed.

You can't push or pressure. That will sabotage your efforts. Even *a single remark* on your part that indicates pressure or exasperation can destroy *any progress* that has been made so far. You must be vigilant and exemplary. You must walk the talk of impeccable acceptance and good manners if you want her to respond in kind.

Simultaneously don't have any expectations. Have good intentions but no expectations. Understand that *"winning" isn't getting your way!* Winning is both of you feeling good, loving and close to each other. Create a safe-space with patience and no pressure. This helps it not feel "creepy" to her.

Next, figure out your intention. What is your "why?" Why do you want to do this? Make sure you do your homework first. You must be able to clearly explain *why you want to do it.* What is your end goal or highest vision for what could happen afterwards? For example, "My

141

intention is that it'll make us both feel really amazing and bring us closer together." Being able to explain your *why* gives her something that she can say "yes" to and helps her to both: a) know you deeper and, b) understand you better! *This is very important!* If you don't do this then she may only have her preconceived notions to go on.

You want to try to fill her mind with the wonderful possibilities instead. Tell her why it's important to you, what your likes and dislikes are and what your commitments are. When you can explain "why," *with deep sharing, vulnerability and authenticity...* she will be more receptive. To help figure out your "why," ask yourself questions like these:

- Why do I want to do this with her?
- Why *now*?
- What is in it for the both of us?
- What is in it for her?
- What is in it for me personally?
- Do I want it to bring us closer together in some way? What way(s)?

Then you must set the stage and give her a frame of reference before you tell her. This is how you figure out where/when/how to tell her. If you just blurt it out, you may trigger a shock reaction in her. That engages her fight or flight nervous system. Even just being radically-honest all by itself can trigger a shock reaction! It's like being naked. If you are in a relationship where emotional nakedness is not acceptable, by suddenly being emotionally naked it will be shocking and unacceptable. That shock reaction separates and distances her from her ability to feel into what you are proposing.

By setting the stage and giving her a frame of reference, you alert her to what is coming, which gives her time to adjust her internal landscape to receive the information. *Now* might not be the best time. Maybe she is in the middle of something. Maybe she must do some urgent or important things right now. Maybe her mind is on something else. You want the highest chances of success. To do that you want her full attention. She can't give you her full attention if her mind is elsewhere, so to stack the deck in your favor you must alert her to what is coming and help her understand what it is generally about so that she can get ready to receive it.

No one likes to be sideswiped or caught off guard. This is about being respectful to your partner and about setting the stage so that your invitation can go as well as possible. Honor her ability to focus on you and pick a time that is good to share it. Don't share it when it's a bad time, but don't let it go for more than a day or two. Let me repeat that. Don't let it go for more than a day or two. A week is too long. Letting it go for more than a day or two is letting yourself be a doormat. You need to stand up for yourself while also being respectful that any given single moment might not be an appropriate time for her to be receptive. But surely you can make a time within a day or two that will be appropriate.

If you can never find a time to bring it up then either

your partner is completely closed, you are telling yourself too much bullshit, or you are perceiving your partner's openness and availability incorrectly. Regardless, I advocate that you should take the leap and bring it up.

The next step is to try to get her into a place of empathy. To increase our chances of being well received it is of the utmost importance that we try to elicit an empathetic response in her. This means that we want to get her in an energetic state where she is sensitive to us and feeling what it is like to be us. If she is in a state where she doesn't give a shit about what you feel, then your chances of a good outcome are zero. However, if you can get her in a place where she is feeling openness and love for you then your chances of a good outcome are much higher.

We do this by being transparent and telling her what our fears are. By being honest, forthcoming and authentic about what is happening and *what we are afraid of* (about telling her this desire) we hopefully can foster an empathetic reaction in her. For example, if I say to my girlfriend, "I'm afraid to tell you this thing that I would like to try sexually with you because I'm afraid you will get mad at me or judge me," I increase the likelihood that she will soften to me and not get mad at me or judge me.

Naming our fear of a negative reaction tends to counteract her having that negative reaction because if she still reacts in that negative way after you tell her the thing that you want to tell her, then she demonstrates that your fear is justified in the first place. Again, we are talking about increasing chances of success here. There are no guarantees. You need to understand that hearing what someone wants to do to you sexually *is an uncommon thing to talk about*. If she has an emotional reaction *nothing is wrong*. Don't flinch or apologize or take it back. Apologizing makes it sound like it's bad. Just *let it be*. Just let her have her time to settle then ask her what she *thinks*. Since it's an uncommon thing to talk about, she may not have had anyone speak to her like this before. You then have a chance to role-model good communication and how to share deeply and authentically to her. There is no guarantee that she will respond positively, but role-modeling it increases your odds.

Here are the phases of this strategy of bringing up your desire:

1) Make her aware that there is something you want to *invite her* to do with you sexually and ask her when a good time is to have the conversation (in case this moment is not a good time).

2) When you get to the time to ask her, tell her a few of your reasons why you are afraid of bringing it up in the first place. Be real and vulnerable. Be courageous.

3) Then tell her your intention and ideal outcome for bringing it up. Explain why it is important to you to do this sexual thing with her and what you hope it will do for you both.

4) Tell her that even if she doesn't want to do it, it's ok! You just want to start *a conversation about it without putting any pressure on her to do it*.

145

5) Tell her your desire. Ask her what you want to invite her to do with you. The key here is not to put too much "story" in it. If it takes you more than a few sentences to ask her then there is too much "story" in it. Keep it short and direct.

6) Don't take it back. Don't apologize. Don't try to fix it if she reacts negatively. Just let her have her time and reaction and process, and then ask her what she *thinks*. If she has a strong emotional reaction tell her that you see that she is *feeling* the way she is feeling but ask her to *tell you what her thoughts are* so that you can have a conversation because you want to engage her in a rational conversation about it. If needed, reassure her that nothing is going to happen unless you both agree. It just means that you are starting a conversation. That's all.

It often helps to have an example, so let me give you an example of one way this system could be used to bring up a desire to try having anal sex with her.

"There is something that I would like to do with you sexually that I would like to have a conversation about with you. If now isn't a good time then we can do it later, but if now is a good time then I'd like to talk about it now. If now isn't a good time, then when can we talk when you'll be free to have some time to talk and really hear me?

So there is this thing that I would love to do with

you sexually, but I am afraid to bring it up with you because I'm afraid that you'll judge me negatively and that by bringing it up you might think I just think about sex or that I'm a pervert, but I want to share this invitation with you because I want you to be the person who I get to explore my sexual fantasies and edges with!

See, I want us to have next-level sexual fun with each other, and to me sex is an amazing way to explore creativity and connection, and there are lots of sexual things that I've never done that I'd love to do some time. So, I want to see if you are open to having a conversation, and I want us to be completely honest and real with each other, and I feel like I need to share what my fantasies are with you so that you know who I really am inside.

The thing that I want to invite you to do is to try letting me have anal sex with you in a way that makes us both feel amazing, respected and honored, starting slowly and carefully to make sure that it never hurts or feels uncomfortable.

What do you think?"

This method of bringing up a desire is very similar to the system of bringing up a difficult conversation and saying the unsaid that we covered in Chapter 4. Notice the similarities. When you learn this type of approach it will serve you in many areas of your life in many different relationships.

You can use it to bring up your fantasies too. By making it OK to discuss your fantasies together, you unlock a potential world of play and pleasure that otherwise remains forever unobtainable. The more you ask for what you want and share your fantasies, the easier it becomes to talk about these things. They can get exponentially easier and easier until the point where it's no longer a weird or awkward conversation and simply becomes an honest sharing of your thoughts and feelings.

To better help you to really "get" this concept, I've built a worksheet for you to use to work out a script to ask for what you really want. See Appendix B in the back of this book for a worksheet that you can use (as many times as you need) to figure out how to bring up the things that you want to do sexually with your partner. It's one thing to read a chapter and think you "get" the concept, but it is altogether more powerful to "cement" the concept by doing the work. It's the difference between theoretical understanding and practice. I encourage you to do the worksheet to really "get" the concepts so you can walk the talk.

Section 5:

Improve Your Sex Technique

Chapter 26: Lasting Longer in Bed

Let's learn about ejaculation control as a technique for lasting longer in bed. Statistically speaking, men tend to orgasm within two to seven minutes of intercourse. That's simply not long enough for most women to reach orgasm, and in order to improve your love life and relationship you need to be able to satisfy your partner. That means being able to last longer in bed than the average guy. Trust me, you want your partner to think of you as the best lover she's ever had, to brag to her friends about how awesome you are in bed and to feel amazing because you simply rock her world and give her tons of real juicy orgasms!

There are lots of techniques and approaches to ejaculation control. One popular today that I do not recommend is tantric ejaculation avoidance. They teach that it's possible to separate ejaculation from orgasm, which basically means that you can experience the pleasure of orgasm without actually having semen come out of your cock.

The big problem with it from my perspective and experience (and the main reason I don't teach it) is that it can be hard to learn, difficult to master and may contribute to prostate health problems in older men. Many men spend years trying to master it, and anything that you try to master for years can cause feelings of failure and frustration for not being able to succeed. Also, biologically and physiologically orgasms are required for male reproductive health! Prostate health in men over 40 literally depends on having frequent and regular ejaculations. Basically you "use it or you lose it" as the saying goes, and if you don't ejaculate at least once every week or two the prostate can harden, becoming more rigid and less flexible, which can result in prostate cancer. That is a thing that you absolutely want to avoid at all costs.

So, I recommend simple techniques that are easy to learn and quick to implement and that will pay immediate benefits to you. First a little context. Let's define premature ejaculation as ejaculating at any point before *both* of you are completely satisfied. This means that we need to reorient your brain to shift your focus from "getting laid" to "having sex."

The way I use these terms is this: Getting laid is having intercourse and having an orgasm, usually in two to seven minutes like most men, but having sex means enjoying a wide variety of sexual activity and connection without your or her orgasm necessarily being the goal. For example, in this way of looking at it, having sex can encompass oral sex, making out, hand jobs, and all types of penetration for pleasure, while getting laid tends to just be about a fuck that makes the man come, and then the festivities are over. By shifting your focus in this way, you open the door in your mind to longer, more explorative and playful sex rather than "wham bam thank you mam" ...which usually leaves the woman unsatisfied and thinking of you as inconsiderate and only caring about your own needs.

You want her to think of you as a conscious cock, and

for you to be that you must take power and control over your orgasm and come when you decide to come rather than when your penis wants you to. It totally happens that we mean to last longer but reach the point of no return and lose control. That's OK, and it's to be expected when training yourself to get control over your ejaculation. Don't sweat it. Just acknowledge it, think about it afterwards and think about what you could do differently next time so that it doesn't happen again.

Integrate your insights. Be strategic and improve your approach. Don't use orgasm to avoid emotional intimacy with your partner either. It's better to have a good emotional connection, a long sex session and no orgasm than it is to have a shallow emotional connection, short sex session and quick ejaculation. If you just want a quick orgasm, I say that in terms of improving your relationship it's better to masturbate by yourself than to use her to achieve what you want. For women the connection is the most important part, not the orgasm, so slow down, open up and let yourself connect with her while having sex.

Here's how to do it. First start by having a little conversation with her. Tell her that you want to make love for longer in general, that you want to not have orgasms right away and ask her if she could please support and assist you by not making you come so fast. Enlist her help and ask for her support, understanding and patience to help you make this improvement in your sex life. Tell her you both need to change what you are doing because it takes two and that you can't do this without any help from her. Get her to agree that "stop" means "stop immediately," and that she'll stop moving if you say stop.

Next let me explain to you the zero to ten scale of male arousal. Think of it like this. Zero is zero arousal. Completely flaccid. Ten is having an orgasm. Nine is the point of no return. Eight is the spot just before the point of no return--it is your last chance to stop. OK, ready for the secret to ejaculation control? It's this: keep your state of arousal in the five to seven range. When you get up to seven or eight you must change what you are doing to keep you from getting to nine: the point of no return.

That's it! It's simple, *but that doesn't mean it's easy*, so let me show you my method for staying in the five to seven range. First understand that deep thrusting with long slides into her and long slides out of her will escalate you towards 10 very quickly, and that side to side motions where you aren't moving in and out will not stimulate you very much, but they will stimulate her very well.

A major key in being able to last longer in intercourse is not pounding her or being pounded by her, but instead being inside of her with smaller motions that are less stimulating to you. Deep thrusting is not the best sex technique. It does not create the best pleasure for women because most of her sensory nerves are in her clitoris not her vagina! Sure, women may moan and cry a lot during deep thrusting, but that is often because it is *more intense*, not because it is more pleasurable.

I really want you to understand this distinction between intense and pleasurable. Imagine you are at a concert of the music that you find the most beautiful in the world. Just hearing it live is a delicious pleasurable thing to you and it carries you away in delight. Now imagine that they turn up the volume so much that you must cover your ears. Sure, the music is still pleasurable, but now it is so intense that it kind of detracts from the pleasure and actually hurts a bit.

Don't get me wrong. Deep thrusting and hard pounding have their place in conscious cock sex, but not when you are trying to last longer in bed. I recommend reserving the intense deep thrusting and pounding for the end when you are ready to come and she is ready for you to come, not during the first five to 10 minutes of lovemaking.

Remember that most of her pleasure nerves are in her clitoris and the entrance to her vagina, not deep inside nor in the vaginal wall. So, to stimulate her better have your penis deep inside of her and move it side to side, like left to right or front to back. When you do this while your pubic bone is pressed against her pubic bone, your pubic bone will stimulate her clitoral head and the sides of your cock will stimulate her clitoral bulbs on the left and right sides of her vaginal opening. It is deliciously pleasurable for her, not intense, won't risk hurting her cervix like deep pounding can do, and is not very stimulating for you so you will be able to last a long time without getting to eight or nine.

To play with this, I recommend the yab yum position. Yab yum means "union," and in this position you sit with your legs crossed (or extended out or on a chair) and she sits on top of you with her legs wrapped around you.

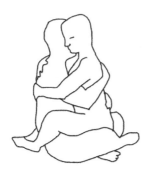

With her on top of you like this, she can gyrate her hips and move side-to-side and you can't do deep thrusting. It puts you face-to-face and your hearts close together--which fosters the connection that women crave and the long lovemaking that is usually required for her to relax and open deeply to pleasure.

Even men who normally come in under five minutes often find that the first time they do yab yum with their partner they can last half an hour or more, and that the experience of lovemaking with their partner is deeper, more fulfilling and more satisfying. Many report that after that long they no longer even care about having an orgasm, and that their partner often experiences so much pleasure and relaxation that she has multiple orgasms! A shift occurs, from taking pleasure only from his orgasm to taking pleasure in being deeply pleasing to his partner. While helping you delay orgasm it simultaneously helps her get closer to orgasm.

That said, whenever you experience an escalation bringing you close to eight or nine, whether it is during yab yum or deep thrusting or any other position or technique, first off *stop completely* and *breathe deep*. Stop your motion all together and tell her "*stop*" if necessary. Take control if she doesn't help you and pull out immediately and squeeze down hard and long on your PC muscle until the spike in penis arousal passes and subsides.

I can't say it enough to breathe deeply repeatedly and squeeze down hard on your PC muscle to avoid falling off the cliff of the point of no return. If you can simply *slow down* your strokes' speed and reduce the amount you are going in and out to a slow shallow in and out then great, but you may need to change your position entirely to one that gives you less powerful stimulation, like yab yum. You can't expect to just fast fuck in doggy style and never come (like guys in porn movies). Many of them are on Viagra which gives them artificial superhuman sex powers. They aren't real or to be believed nor idolized.

What you want is to draw out the pleasure until she fills to overflowing with pleasure or orgasms. Then choose when you want to release and ejaculate. Don't make her orgasms your goal, however. That will disconnect you from her because you are focused on something that may or may not happen. Instead make *her pleasure* your goal and draw out the pleasure if you both enjoy it.

Now, in addition to slowing down, breathing deep, stopping and switching positions to something less stimulating like yab yum, there are lots of other things you can also do to calm down to the five to seven range if you find yourself at eight or nine. One powerful technique is to change what you are doing. Stop having intercourse and either go down on her or give her a hand job or make out with her or emotionally connect and chat for a while or give her a massage or get out a vibrator or spank her or something else that she likes that doesn't involve stimulating your penis. Switch it up for a while and then go back to intercourse after you have cooled down a lot!

Gauge her arousal level visually and tell her that you want to stop having intercourse and do something else for a little while so that you don't come yet and tell her what you'd like to do and ask her what she'd enjoy. For example, offer her oral, a hand job, massage, dildo, vibrator, kissing, chocolate and let her choose! Say that you want to continue with intercourse in a little while when you've cooled down, but be okay if it doesn't happen! You can always give yourself an orgasm later, but you can't manufacture deep erotic sexual connection with her on the spot, and if you just let yourself come then that would end the deep sexual connection in a moment, preventing you from reaching the heights that you could reach if you continue to pleasure her!

Understand that you may need to give up your orgasms and the pleasure you derive from them for a while in order to gain more control. It's giving up short-term superficial pleasure for deeper long-term satisfaction, and it's totally worth it. You can always masturbate to have an orgasm, so it's fine to play with not having an orgasm at all during sex with your partner in order to improve your control and her respect for your ability to control it!

That's my conscious cock system for ejaculation control in a nutshell. For a deeper dive into mastering these techniques, watch my free three-video mini course. Find it in the recommended resources section of Appendix A. If you have any questions, comments, successes or failures please share them in the Facebook group.

Chapter 27: Hand Jobs

In my experience most people think that hand jobs are just for guys, but that couldn't be further from the truth. Hand jobs are just pleasing your partner with your hands and that means hand jobs are for women too!

Hands can often be the best tool for the job because they are super dexterous and sensitive, and they can grip, squeeze and trace as well as insert fingers--not to mention the fact that we have two of them so we can alternate between hands and give contrasting motions at the same time! Since they are much more nimble, agile and sensitive, hands are much more capable of producing orgasm for a woman than a cock is. So if you want to improve your relationship then give your woman more hand jobs in ways that make her hot and craving more!

First off understand that communication is essential. You must watch her body language and listen to her audible signals. Ask her to give you feedback. Ask, "Is this good?" and "Do you like it when I do it this way?" And if you really want to be the best then ask her to show you how she likes to touch herself or be touched. Then copy her pressure, rhythm and motion as closely as you can. See Appendix D at the back of this book for a helpful exercise for this.

Often women will like a light, sensitive and delicate touch on the outside lips to begin with--to wake up the area and get her warmed up. Don't just go straight to her clit unless she is already heated up or you know for a fact (perhaps by having asked her) that she wants it. Make sure that your fingernails are cut short, hangnails are clipped, and you have sanded or filed down any hard edges. You want your hands to be soft and supple. And make sure to use a lubricant. I recommend a silicone lube like Eros Bodyglide or Swiss Navy. A little bit goes a long way and they last a very long time and don't get sticky (but be sure not to use a silicone sex toy afterwards because the silicone lube will bond to it like glue and wreck it).

So, start with the outer labia, tracing and seductively caressing them up and down from above her clit to down below her vaginal opening. Caress the inner labia also and cup her entire vulva. Just being held can feel amazing, and while you cup and hold her you can kiss her and press gently with your palm and move your hand in small circular motions to wake up the whole area.

The idea is to start outside and work your way in. Most women don't enjoy a finger just jabbing in and out hard and fast. You must think subtle, sensuous and intoxicating rather than mindless jamming in and out. Circle with a well-lubed finger around her clitoral head and her vaginal opening without sliding inside. Roll the clitoral shaft gently between your thumb and forefinger. Vary your pressure from light to medium to firm, asking her what she likes the best and watching her body language like her taking deep breaths, her belly rising and falling, and if she grinds her hips down towards you or groans, you know you are on the right track.

Let her be your guide and set your intention to follow her as best as you can until you understand what she likes and then work that for a while. When she's good and hot, then slowly slip one finger inside her and pause to simply feel how delicious she feels wrapped around your finger. It's extremely erotic and satisfying to have your finger in her life center, isn't it? After grounding with her in stillness for a few moments, then begin to use circular motions and a "come hither" motion rather than an in-and-out motion. The in-and-out doesn't do much to activate her pleasure centers like her clitoral legs, G-spot, A-spot and kundalini spot, but a come hither motion, circular, up-and-down, and side-to-side motions do. Think like a lesbian, not a guy.

If you can lay her on her back and take one hand to rub and massage her clit while the other hand has a finger inside of her massaging her from the inside, you will really drive her wild. When she's opened enough that she's not tight on just one finger any more, slowly slide a second or third inside so that she has a pleasant sensation of tightness on your fingers while you massage her pussy.

Hands can get tired if you are doing a fast and vigorous motion, so take breaks and shift to something else like giving her head or playing with a toy like a vibrator for a while. Don't wear yourself out and don't be a mindless pile driving machine on her either. You can increase her arousal by going in cycles, by building up the intensity of pressure and velocity until you get to a fast commanding pace, but then slow down again and let both of you recover for a while and switch to slower more languid strokes, and then repeat the process. You can repeat this until you level her up to the point of orgasm, multiple orgasm, whole body orgasms, and ejaculations. You literally can bring her to the point of being a quivering screaming explosion of pleasure and catharsis, so be sure that you *stay present* with her and don't drop her or draw back. She's trusting that you are going to carry her through the experience to the other side, so be there for her and stay with her consciously through the whole journey, whatever happens. Gauge her and follow and track her and adjust what you are doing to support her where she is at every moment. You are giving her a gift here so hold a high intention to see her through the journey of her pleasure to the point where she is finished.

Your loving devotion to her pleasure and experience will make her more giving to you in return, so it is a fantastic positive feedback loop. Hand jobs are a great way to have hot sex and intimacy without needing to have intercourse, which means that they are also a great form of birth control if she's in the fertile part of her monthly cycle. Also, you can do a hand job through or underneath clothes, which means that you can have great sex without even needing to get naked, which is awesome for quickies and hot sex in places where it's not possible or appropriate to take your clothes off.

For a great and completely sexually explicit instructional video on hand jobs for both men and women, I recommend that you check out Tristan Taormino's *Ultimate Guide to Hand Jobs* video. If you have any questions, comments, successes or failures to share please post them in the Facebook group.

Chapter 28: Oral Sex (Cunnilingus)

The terms "oral sex," "going down," "eating out," and "dining at the Y" all refer to the act of cunnilingus, which means licking the vulva in Latin. Whether you are a cunnilingus Jedi, have tried it and didn't like it or have never tried it, this chapter is going to cover a lot and you'll probably learn something that will improve your sex life. We'll cover the benefits to a man who goes down on a woman, the dangers, concerns, techniques and some positions.

There are a lot of benefits of cunnilingus, and they are not all for the woman! Going down on a woman is an honoring and empowering practice that helps a man to increase his stamina. Her sexual fluids contain great hormones and components that may help the health and immunity of the man's prostate. Her vaginal flora is full of probiotics, and probiotics (like kombucha, yogurt and other fermented foods) can improve the man's digestive health and function. For her, cunnilingus triggers the release of oxytocin and endorphins. These hormones are known to reduce pain, strengthen the immune system, lower blood pressure, fight heart disease and cancer, counteract depression and elevate her mood! Not only that but emotionally she experiences an improved trust with you because you demonstrate that you are interested in what feels good to her and accept and love her body.

With all benefits come dangers too, and as with any

body fluid, sexually transmitted infections and non-sexual infections like yeast infections can be transmitted from vulva to mouth and vice versa. These can all be mitigated by using a barrier shield, like a sheet of saran wrap or a dental dam to block the transmission of fluids between the two of you. A side benefit of this is that it also blocks her from feeling your facial hair if you have a mustache or beard, and you don't get any pubic hair stuck in your teeth or on your tongue. Another danger of cunnilingus is that you might give her an infection by transferring harmful bacteria from her anus to her vaginal area since they are close together. Never lick her anus and then lick her vulva! Also, if you have a cold sore on your lip or gums *do not* go down on her! Cold sores are a form of the Herpes virus, and you could give your oral herpes to her pussy!

As well as these potential dangers there are also concerns that you should address. Many women experience self-consciousness about someone going down on them. Much of this can come from worries about hygiene, which can be addressed by talking about them and washing and cleaning. Ask her what would make her feel more comfortable--like maybe taking a shower first, trimming her pubic hair, turning off the lights, putting on some perfume... whatever she wants. There is no need to douche however, as it just throws off her natural vaginal balance and can lead to problems like yeast or bacterial infections.

I highly recommend that when you get ready to go down on her you smell her vulva gently first. Every woman is different, and any specific woman changes daily--and you are not expected to always like the way she smells or tastes! You don't have to be a non-feeling robot who will do anything! The reverse is true for her also. She doesn't always have to like the way you smell or taste.

See if you like the way she smells before you go down on her. Nuzzle into her pubic mound. Many guys find they *love* the way she smells, and it makes them want to taste her. A few little tastes with the tongue will tell you if you want to go further, but if she doesn't smell good to you don't force yourself to go down on her! She might have a yeast infection or bacterial infection and not even know it. Be kind, be gentle and share with her that you'd rather do something else because something doesn't smell quite right and maybe she might want to go to the gynecologist for an exam. Feel free to not say it right then but wait until the next day so that you don't kill the moment. The idea here is not to be a jerk nor to make her feel self-conscious, but rather to be a *health ally* with her and support her in her sexual health. If she smells good or bad to you, follow your instinct and communicate gently and respectfully with her.

Now let's move on to technique, assuming that yes, you do want to go down on her and have addressed the STI and health precautions. First, some don'ts. Don't go down on her after eating spicy food or power mints or mouthwash, as you could burn her. Don't spit on her to lube her up nor blow into her vagina. Don't bite her at all (unless she's asked you and you've talked about how she likes it). Don't just flick her clit endlessly, and don't lick her anus and then lick her vulva, even if she just washed. You don't want to transfer any bacteria from the anal area to the vulva! Don't expect an orgasm and don't go down on her as a means of just getting to have intercourse with her... that's an inauthentic thing to do. Do it for the *joy and pleasure of connecting with her in this very intimate way*. Do it for her pleasure and your own.

Pay attention to her body language, the sounds she makes, and listen to anything she tells you. Moaning is good but squirming or pulling away or making sounds of discomfort are signals that you aren't doing things the way that she enjoys. Let her be your guide. Every woman is different and any single woman's likes and enjoyments change over time and with her mood or state of mind or point in her monthly cycle. What worked on her yesterday may not be enjoyable for her today, so if in doubt, *ask her* what she wants in that moment. See Appendix D at the back of this book for a helpful exercise for this. If she is pressing into you or gyrating in some way, try to sync up with her motion because she is showing you what rhythm and motion she likes.

That said, in general it's good to start slow and supple and arouse her body by massage and caressing her belly and breasts and thighs but avoid touching the clit until she's very turned on. There is no need to penetrate her with anything during oral sex. Just the licking and kissing can be more than enough to be amazingly pleasurable to her. However, if she is super turned on and craves having you or having something inside her, it can be fantastic to her to have your finger massage her G-spot while your mouth kisses and licks her clit. The key is to enjoy *each stroke* of your tongue, *each kiss* and touch of your lips. Be *slow* and don't rush it. The key to her enjoyment of you giving her oral sex is in its gentleness. Don't have a sharp five o'clock shadow and expect it to feel good to her to have your razor-sharp face touching her soft bits. Be soft and supple when you love her down there.

Some specific techniques to try include licking from the fourchette (which is the area between her anus and vagina) up to the clitoral hood and shaft in long slow strokes. Just don't lick her anus and then her vagina! When she's super turned on, and her pussy lips are fully engorged then lick her clit, try vertically and also horizontally back and forth. Try circles around it. Try deeper slower pressure and faster lighter pressure and ask her what she likes best if you can't tell from her body language. Also try *very* gently sucking on her clit, pulling it gently into your mouth and sucking on it. See if she likes it. While doing all of this occasionally caress her breasts and play with her nipples. The simultaneous pleasure of clit stimulation from oral sex with nipple stimulation with the hands can easily make many women come!

If she is super well-aroused, then try slowly and gently inserting a well lubed finger and make a come hither motion to stimulate her G-spot. If she doesn't feel tight around your finger, slowly insert two or three fingers as needed to create a feeling of fullness or tightness. Lick her clit while making a come hither motion with your finger. *Don't* just jab your finger in and out, but rather make slow come hither motions that touch and massage her G-spot while simultaneously licking her clitoral head. If in doubt, *ask her*, and remember where her sensory hotspots are and touch and massage them in ways that will be pleasurable to her.

The most important thing is to switch it up in the beginning and pay attention to what she responds to and then pick what she likes best and focus on it. Be consistent and don't change your rhythm or motion because it can make her lose the orgasm. Many women take many minutes of consistent clit licking before they will reach orgasm, so be prepared to show some stamina and really show up for her so that she has the time it takes her to relax into the pleasure and open to her orgasms. Harder isn't better. Faster isn't better. Connected, aware and responsive is better.

If your mouth or tongue ever get too tired, switch up what you are doing to use your fingers or a dildo or a vibrator or whatever she tells you she'd like you to do to her. Don't wear yourself out. Refocus, check-in and take care of yourselves! It's a good idea to come up for air occasionally to give yourself a break and look her deeply in the eyes to punctuate this very intimate act! Vary what you are doing and then go back down on her when you are ready to continue.

The 69 position is great to give you both simultaneous stimulation. It's wonderful to lay on your sides with a pillow or her leg under your head for support. Make sure that you are comfortable and don't stress out your neck or body! If you must lift your head up to reach her pussy, you will wear out your neck muscles and be sore after. It's worth it to get a pillow or two or adjust your position to get the right amount of support and lift. Every bit of attention you put on comfort will result in you both being able to relax deeper into more pleasure.

You can also lay on your back while she kneels over your face and lowers herself down to your mouth. This is more empowering for her to control the amount of pressure and tease you.

She also can get down on all fours so you can lick her from behind and she can lay on her back and put her hips and butt on a pillow to make it easier on your neck. Regardless, pick a comfortable position for both of you so that you don't stress your body.

With all this, remember to ask her first if she'd like you to go down on her. She might not want you to. If she says no, then just respect her desire and drop it. Don't try to push it on her, but you can simply ask her if there is anything else that she would like you to do to her instead.

I encourage you to talk with your partner about cunnilingus and find out what she likes and doesn't like, what her concerns and worries are, and to ask her how you can improve your sex life with cunnilingus. Let her be your guide and explore the wonderful world of oral sex together. Again, see Appendix D at the back of this book for a helpful exercise for this, and please post any questions, comments, successes or challenges in the Facebook group.

Chapter 29: Intercourse

We've made it to the coup de grace of the Conscious Cock owner's manual... intercourse! Now we bring it all together and will be turning you into a sex God who really knows how to fuck a woman in a way that should both get her off and make her think of you as the best lover she's ever had. We want to create an experience that makes her absolutely hunger for you - one that makes her want to tell her friends what an amazing lover you are!

Note: We are only going to be talking about vaginal intercourse here. We are not going to get into anal sex. Plenty of guys want to fuck their woman in the ass, but I consider it an advanced technique that I'm not going to cover in this 101-level book. You have enough to master with just the clitoris, vagina, G-spot, A-spot and cervix right now. Let's save the ass for after you've mastered the pussy because it is a completely different approach.

First let's talk about the benefits and dangers of intercourse. Well-done sex increases intimacy and attachment, eases stress, improves sleep, balances hormone levels, boosts libido, improves bladder control and lowers blood pressure! It makes you both feel more connected and happier when done right. But there are dangers too. It can lead to unwanted pregnancy, cause urinary tract infections and yeast infections and can transmit sexually transmitted infections. No one likes to deal with health problems in their nether regions, and an unwanted pregnancy is one hell of a mood killer for your sex life!

So be smart. Get tested so that you know for sure if you do or don't have any STIs. Take a shower and wash your cock and balls with a good amount of regular soap, not the antibacterial stuff with harsh scents that can cause irritation. Get properly fitting condoms if you are concerned about giving or getting an STI or causing an unwanted pregnancy.

If you have a big cock, then get the plus-sized condoms. If you are average or small, then get the condoms that say "slim" or "slim fit" or "thin" because they will stay on better. Brush your teeth and trim your nails. Gargle with mouthwash, wash off any body odor, and if you shave regularly then make sure you don't have a rough five o'clock shadow. You want to be both delicious to her senses and clean so that you don't cause her a UTI or yeast infection which would be really annoying for her and ultimately reduce her availability for sex with you!

Let's get your mindset set right to make intercourse the best it can possibly be. Think about the name "Intercourse." Think of it as one course of an extravagant multi-course meal in a fine restaurant. In conscious lovemaking there can be many more courses after intercourse.

Foreplay starts with awareness and planning. For her to open to you fully so that you have a chance of turning her into an insatiable sex Goddess who just wants to worship your cock, and have you fuck her brains out, you need to address the concerns that are on her mind so that she can relax! Things like privacy, tiredness, cleanliness, STI protection and birth control can all be a huge mood killer for her. If you address them up front, then maybe she can relax into delicious passion.

Also set your attitude right. Make it all about giving her an invitation to pleasure. Don't try to convince her to have sex with you. Don't pressure her. Pressure and convincing are not sexy.

The conscious cock way to do it is to make her hungry for you by being a considerate and empowered lover who takes care of all the little details so that she can really let go fully in trust and pleasure. Make your goal *mutual pleasure*, not your orgasm! Aim to draw out the delicious pleasure as long as possible. Don't make her orgasm your goal either. *Make the pleasure the goal.* If you make her orgasm your goal, then you might create a situation where she feels like she needs to fake an orgasm.

If you just make her pleasure your goal and stay focused on her body language and vocal cues, then you will stay connected with what is really happening for her. Listen for any sounds of discomfort or the appearance that she pulls away. If you see either of those then immediately stop what you are doing and ask her if that is hurting and then change to something else that won't hurt her. Also set your goal that you won't have an orgasm for at least 15 minutes to half an hour, and then after that that you won't come until you are both ready for it. You want her to be so hot and bothered that she is literally craving your semen so

173

that when you eventually come, she is fiending for it and screaming, "Yes, yes, yes!!!" Let me assure you that there is nothing hotter!

Let's move on to technique. First of all, don't even think of having intercourse until she is completely aroused and fully turned on. Use her level of lubrication as a guide (unless she has told you or you have observed that her level of lubrication is not a reliable indicator of her level of arousal). Aside from that case, if she isn't wet enough for you to easily enter then she isn't turned on enough yet! It's as simple as that. To get her turned on you must arouse her mind, her emotions and her body. Remember the top down approach? Just turning on one of them won't do it. You want her to be so hungry to be filled by your cock that she'll literally pounce on you!

To turn on her mind you can tell her what you'd like to do to her or with her. To turn on her heart you can tell her how you feel about her and what you appreciate about her. To turn on her body think massage, making out, caresses and all forms of foreplay that we have covered.

Now listen. There's one thing that you really need to understand. Don't just shove it in and pile drive your cock into her cervix. Enter slowly and retract slowly halfway at first. It's not a race to your orgasm! It's an enjoyment of...every...single...second of sensation and connection. Draw it out. Make the anticipation build ever higher and higher.

The way that women are built anatomically is such that

just in and out motions don't really do much for them until they are at maximum levels of arousal, and even then you have to hit the right deep erogenous zones by the cervix and A-spot, and even that is hit or miss for the same woman based on what point she is in her cycle. So, in-and-out isn't the best way to please her body. Think more side-to-side, circular motions, up-and-down, back-and-forth and rhythm... not pounding. Lots of women are hurt by their man just being a raging bull, and you want her to love how you fuck her, not to be hurt by it. Think about her anatomy - the location and shape of her clitoris and have intercourse in ways that stimulate it rather than ignore it.

While having intercourse monitor your arousal level. On a zero to ten scale, keep it in the five to seven range so you don't come. If or when you get close to climax, *pull out immediately* and start giving her a hand job or oral sex or kissing and hugging. Then continue the intercourse after your arousal has lessened. Switch to a less stimulating position and breathe deeply. Holding your breath and pounding in a very stimulating position will just make you come before you are both ready.

When you are ready to come and you can tell that she is ready for you to come, ask her where she'd like you to come! She might want you to come inside her or on her boobs, or in her mouth or in the condom (if you are wearing one) or onto a towel or washcloth. She may not enjoy a wet spot on the bed either, so have a towel on hand to catch it or wipe it up. If you don't ask, then you will never know! If your give it to her how and where she wants it, she's going to love it and love how you respect her desires and preferences.

That said, remember: don't make your orgasm the goal. Be the amazing man who is big enough that he doesn't need to have an orgasm to enjoy having sex. You can always go masturbate later. Stay in the moment with her. Stay connected and track her experience and enjoyment more than your desire to "get off." It shows her that you value her, and that tends to make her more open and willing to fuck you in amazing ways.

If you do come then take a minute to recuperate, and then continue to make love to her for a while longer! This will drive her absolutely wild if she is super turned on and will set you apart from 99% of guys who would just turn over and fall asleep. If you used a condom withdraw and pull off the condom, wipe off your cock and put a fresh one on to continue, or make love to her by using your hands or going down on her or do some massage. *Draw out her pleasure* and help her to come down gently or wait through your recuperation period and then have intercourse with her again. Most men find that after they've had one orgasm and recovered that then if they have intercourse again, they can last ten times longer!

To really seal the lovemaking session with a beautiful ending, afterwards tell her three things that you really enjoyed and that were hot for you. For example, "I loved it when you did that thing with your hands." And, if you love her, tell her so! Using your words is one of the best ways to have sex mentally and emotionally, and it cements in her that she is safe with you and that you are congruent. Then ask her what her favorite part/technique/moment was!

In all of this, don't wear yourself out. If you get tired or are working so hard that you are dripping in sweat, you aren't doing it right. Slow down and remember to focus on pleasure. Switch positions so that you don't wear your body out. Take turns being in the driver's seat. Lovemaking is all about taking turns being the active partner and the receiving partner.

The Missionary position is great for the beginning. It gives you both full frontal contact, and it can be both amazingly pleasurable and very gentle. Just be extremely conscious not to put all your weight on her so that she can't breathe! Prop yourself up on your elbows so she can breathe.

The Cowgirl position is when you are on your back and she sits on top of you. Cowgirl is great because she's in control. She controls depth and speed and motion while you get the best view and can play with her belly and breasts. It's also harder for you to do much pounding in-and-out motion while in cowgirl, so it can help you to last longer while giving her more pleasure from rocking and gyrating and grinding her clit on your pubic bone. However, be careful that she doesn't ride you too fast and drive you to an eight or nine. Be ready to grab her hips to stop her motion if you need to stop her from making you cum.

The Doggy Style position is awesome for quickies and is best when she is at maximum level of arousal and when you are ready to come. It stimulates deep vaginal erogenous zones like her A-spot and cervix and can lead to epicenter orgasms that are earth shattering for her, but it can be painful if you are really big or she is small or it's the time of her cycle when her cervix is low, so watch her body language and subtle cues to make sure she's fucking loving it, or else ask!

Now that you've got all this kickass information, go practice! Talk to your partner about intercourse and ask her what her favorite and least favorite things about it are. It'll give you tons of actionable information and demonstrates to her that you value her feelings and want to be a good lover to her. Please post your comments, questions and successes and failures in the Facebook group and remember to keep doing your Kegels and fuck your life!

Putting It All Together

Now that we've gone through installing some upgrades, understanding your partner, increasing your sex education and improving the spark in your relationship and sex life, what's next? Honestly these tools and techniques can be practiced for a lifetime. I urge you not to get caught in the trap of thinking that you need to go learn more things. So many people are always seeking and consuming, but the true magic happens when you implement what you've learned through practice.

With all the material that we have covered, you should now have a strong foundation of authenticity from which to interface with your partner. You should understand her better and know how to interact with her in a more empowered manner while simultaneously maintaining your own center and values. And on top of all that you should be better able to get what you really want out of your sex life.

So, to end, I would like to present you with a final exercise that you can use as a springboard to implement and practice all that you have learned so far. I call it the Yes No Maybe exercise. It will show you where you have open doors with your partner through which to walk and explore these concepts and ways of relating. It helps you and your partner learn what sexual activities and experiences you are open to doing together, which ones you would love to try together, and which ones are off-limits to either of you.

It helps you find the overlap of sexual activities that you both want to explore so that you can expand your sexual and erotic playground in a conscious and loving way while respecting each other's preferences and boundaries. It helps you to bypass assumptions that either of you may have about what the other is interested in (or open to) by directly communicating with each other in a pressure-free manner.

Fill one out and have your partner fill one out. If you are interested in trying something, then put a check in the "Yes" column. If you are open to trying it or talking about it then put a check in the "Maybe" column, and if you are not interested in trying it then put a check in the "No" column. Make sure that you are honest in your answers and that you aren't trying to pleasure your partner or answer the way you think she wants you to answer. Be authentic and bold and ask her to do the same.

When you are both done then compare your lists and see what things you both answered "Yes" to, what things either of you answered "No" to, and what things either of you answered "Maybe" to. You will probably be surprised by what you learn about each other. If one of you answered "Yes" to something that the other answered "Maybe" to, then you get to talk about how it could work if you were to try it sometime! If you both answered "Yes" to something, then you can now embrace that activity as something you want to make happen together and talk about the juicy details of how it turns each of you on! If either of you answered "No" to an activity that the other answered "Yes" or "Maybe" to, then you should simply drop the idea of doing that activity and replace it with something that you both answered "Yes" to. The whole idea is to put zero pressure on each other. Instead you should focus on the feeling of getting to know each other more and finding where your interests overlap, and let that overlap define the sexual playground that you explore together.

If there are multiple things in a row (for example "Take a shower / bath / hot tub together"), then you can circle the thing that you most want to do or discuss. Then in the Notes column you can write any clarifications. You can do this exercise once a year (or more or less) to have a "check-in" and see if anything has changed for either of you. Many people find that as they build trust and a sense of exploration in their relationship, they often become more open to things that they previously had put into the "No" column. But this process of expanding and unfolding into our "Yes" can only happen in an atmosphere of trust, support and zero pressure.

Again, fill one out yourself and have your partner fill out the other one. Then compare notes and enjoy talking about the intersections of your interests and desires. Feel free to copy the worksheets so you can use them again at a later time.

Type of activity	Yes	Maybe	No	Notes
Try anal sex (receiving or giving?)				
Try oral sex (receiving or giving?)				
Threesome with a man				
Threesome with a woman				
Same room sex with another couple				
Being tied up / trying fuzzy handcuffs				
Being blindfolded / teased / dominated				
Try spanking (receiving or giving?)				
Playing with a feather / whip / vibrator / strapon				
Forceful and rough sex				
Masturbate in front of you				
Have you masturbate in front of me				
Masturbate in front of each other				
Have phone sex / try sexting				
Find out what kind of porn you like				
Make a porn/erotic video together				
Play with ice cubes / food				
Have sex in the shower				
Watch another couple have sex				
Have sex in a public place / beach				
Go skinny dipping				
Dance together naked				
Have loud sex or have completely silent sex				
Give or get a blow job/hand job while driving				
Go to a strip club together				
Sleep naked together				
Try new sex positions / practice kama sutra				
Have sex on your desk/on the table				
Try swinging / try group sex				
7day / 30day sex challenge				
Do a sexy boudoir photoshoot				
Sex while drunk / high				
Sex in an airplane / on a boat / in a car				
Have sex in a sex swing				
Try tantra				
Try rimming				
Give sensual body massages to each other				
Have sex with only foreplay & no penetration				
Make a naked bodypaint painting together				
Take a shower / bath / hot tub together				
Have sex during her period				
Have sex in front of a mirror				
Have sex in a room lit with candles				
Do it while someone is watching				
Learn / watch pole dancing				
Master g-spot orgasms				
Try prostate massage				
Nipple play				
Learn to have/give female ejaculation				
Learn to have / give multiple orgasms				
Play dress up / try role playing				
Go lingerie shopping together				
Read erotica together				
Share your sexual fantasies with each other				
Try out different lubes/condoms				

Type of activity	Yes	Maybe	No	Notes
Try anal sex (receiving or giving?)				
Try oral sex (receiving or giving?)				
Threesome with a man				
Threesome with a woman				
Same room sex with another couple				
Being tied up / trying fuzzy handcuffs				
Being blindfolded / teased / dominated				
Try spanking (receiving or giving?)				
Playing with a feather / whip / vibrator / strapon				
Forceful and rough sex				
Masturbate in front of you				
Have you masturbate in front of me				
Masturbate in front of each other				
Have phone sex / try sexting				
Find out what kind of porn you like				
Make a porn/erotic video together				
Play with ice cubes / food				
Have sex in the shower				
Watch another couple have sex				
Have sex in a public place / beach				
Go skinny dipping				
Dance together naked				
Have loud sex or have completely silent sex				
Give or get a blow job/hand job while driving				
Go to a strip club together				
Sleep naked together				
Try new sex positions / practice kama sutra				
Have sex on your desk/on the table				
Try swinging / try group sex				
7day / 30day sex challenge				
Do a sexy boudoir photoshoot				
Sex while drunk / high				
Sex in an airplane / on a boat / in a car				
Have sex in a sex swing				
Try tantra				
Try rimming				
Give sensual body massages to each other				
Have sex with only foreplay & no penetration				
Make a naked bodypaint painting together				
Take a shower / bath / hot tub together				
Have sex during her period				
Have sex in front of a mirror				
Have sex in a room lit with candles				
Do it while someone is watching				
Learn / watch pole dancing				
Master g-spot orgasms				
Try prostate massage				
Nipple play				
Learn to have/give female ejaculation				
Learn to have / give multiple orgasms				
Play dress up / try role playing				
Go lingerie shopping together				
Read erotica together				
Share your sexual fantasies with each other				
Try out different lubes/condoms				

Now What?

If you've made it this far, I want to congratulate you! It takes a lot of commitment and courage to embrace changing our awareness. One of the patterns that I see over and over again in men who want to rise is that they consume all this information but nothing really seems to change in their lives. It's because we often think that just having new accurate information is enough for us to make massive change.

Honestly though, it's only the first ingredient! To make lasting meaningful change we also need a few more ingredients. The information opens your awareness, but to actually cement the concepts to make lasting change you need ongoing support. Then when you have a challenge with implementing a concept or when you try something and it doesn't work out as well as you'd like, you can get ongoing guidance to help you refine and focus your technique and mindset to achieve best results.

Beyond that you also need accountability. That's why I've created the Conscious Cock Brotherhood. There we host weekly online men's circles where we have monthly assignments like the "best month of sex ever challenge," and every week you have to check in on the call and share your progress, your successes and your challenges implementing the concepts and working towards your goal. Knowing that you and all the other guys in the group are going to be checking in about your progress on the monthly assignment each week creates accountability and gives you a structure that helps you to make progress and succeed. Without that there is no anchor to force you to do the work, but with it you make serious lasting gains as we all rise *together*.

If you have a question, you bring it to the men's group. If you have an idea that you want feedback on, you bring it to the men's group. If you have a fail or a win or a tough time with a concept, you bring it to the men's group. In addition to giving you ongoing support, accountability and structure, this also gives you something priceless that men desperately need and never get from other men: encouragement.

The other men in the group celebrate your wins with you, tell you when you did a great job and offer you support, advice and perspectives when you want them. We all inevitably feel confused, overwhelmed and like giving up, but with encouragement from other rising men with similar values, you are better able to stay on track and keep going! This creates the final ingredient that is so powerful for our success: community.

In the group each man gets paired up with another man so that we all have a buddy. By doing that the guys get to form deep supportive friendships that they can call on during the week whenever they have something that they want to share or get support with. No longer do they feel alone and alienated! Instead they are messaging each other when they need help or encouragement, they are giving each other support and feedback at the deepest level, and they have a new best friend with whom they can be completely real.

That's what community does. It shows you that you aren't alone in a desert, and as we all share what is *really* going on for us in our lives and relationships, we learn from each other. Most of us have never had healthy sex-positive male role models. Together we offer each other that in the Brotherhood.

It's so hard to create something that you can't see, but if you have good role-models, then you can try on the ways that they do things to see if they work for you. You can copy the ways the other guys are being successful and see if it's a good fit for your life. It's a turbo boost. It gives you energy and inspiration as you experience solidarity with other good rising men.

My deepest wish for you is to have a community of awesome men to support you on your journey and evolution so that you aren't alone. We are all teachers and students, and you have wisdom inside you that is valuable to other men! So read all the books you want and take all the workshops you can, but then get out there and do the work, and the best way I've seen to do it is with ongoing support, accountability, structure, encouragement and community.

If you can't find that in your area or don't know where to look, then I invite you to join a Conscious Cock Brotherhood men's circle. Each group is closed and has the same 8 men each week so that we really get to know each other in a safe container. You can get on the waiting list for the next group on my site, consciouscock.com, and if you have any questions you can schedule a free 30-minute call with me beforehand.

By joining and committing to the process of showing up for one call each week, you'll be supported to make massive change and reach your relationship and sex-life goals. It really catapults your sex-life satisfaction, relationship success and sense of self confidence--as we all move towards mastery and happiness. It gives you a place to share your gifts and learn from other amazing men who are also on a mission to make the world a better place.

Lastly, if this book has benefitted you in some powerful way and helped you to improve your life or relationship then I would like to invite you to leave a 5-star review for this book on Amazon.com and share what helped you so that this book can better reach and help other men in the future!

Appendices

Appendix A – Links

Conscious Cock Brotherhood:
https://consciouscock.com/brotherhood/

Conscious Cock Facebook Group:
https://www.facebook.com/groups/consciouscock/

Recommended Resources:
https://consciouscock.com/resources/

Appendix B – How to Bring It Up

How to Bring Up the Hard Stuff (or Ask for What You Want) Worksheet

Complete this worksheet to help you create a draft of a script that you can use to bring up a difficult topic or something you want to do sexually with someone. Repeat as many times as necessary until you really get a fine point on all the elements.

You can print out the completed script and have it in hand when you talk with the person so that you don't forget anything important. Having it printed out can help you have the courage to say everything, and you can even say, "This is important to me, so I want to make sure I get it right so please bear with me while I read it from this paper that I wrote it on so that I don't forget anything." Really let yourself be honest here. This is first and foremost an exercise to help you get clarity. You don't have to show this worksheet to anyone unless you want to.

A) What is it that you want to bring up? What is the issue that you want to address? Is it a goal? A change? A thing you want to do? A request? A thing you want to ask not to be done anymore? Asking for support? Asking for respect? Alone time? Coming clean about something you did in the past? Is it something that you want to do with her sexually? Something you've never done before? Something you did before but never with her? Is it a change from how you have been doing things? What about it is a turn-on for you? Whatever it is that you want to ask for or bring up to discuss, write it down here. If you aren't exactly sure what it is then allow yourself to chisel away at it until you get a fine point on it. Write it from a few different angles until you feel you can clearly explain to yourself what it is you want to bring up. Use additional paper, as necessary. Then condense it into just one to two sentences and write it into the line numbered "A1" at the bottom of this section.

_____

_____

_____

_____

_____

What I really want to bring up is: (A1)

_____

_____

B) Why are you afraid of bringing it up? What are you afraid will happen if you bring it up? What are you afraid that the person will do (or not do) if you bring it up? Why are you afraid of that? Has it happened before? Is it a pattern of hers? A pattern of yours? Really let yourself be honest about your fears. Don't judge or minimize them. Just give yourself permission to record your fears *as they are*. Freely write as many as you can think of and then pick the top three and write them into the numbered lines at the bottom of this section.

_____

_____

_____

_____

_____

_____

My top three fears about bringing this up are:

B1) _____

B2) _____

B3) _____

C) Ask yourself what is your hope for bringing it up? What is your best-case scenario for how things could go well after you bring it up? If she was to receive it well and be on board with you, what would happen then? What would things look like if she responded as an ally to you? What do you really want to have happen by bringing this up? Do you want it to bring you closer? Do you want it to foster a deeper connection? An atmosphere of sexual playfulness, honesty or radical acceptance? To clear the air so that you can reconnect? To achieve more pleasure in your relationship? To achieve a goal that you've always had? To achieve a sexual fantasy that you've always had? Have a better home life? Freely write as many good outcomes as you can think of that you would love to have happen after bringing this up. Then pick the top three and number them in order of priority, if you can.

_____

_____

_____

_____

My top three hopeful outcomes for bringing this up are:

C1) _____

C2) _____

C3) _____

Now let's compile everything into a script

- So, there is this thing that I need to share with you, but I am afraid to bring it up with you because...

\<enter B1 here\> _____

_____, and

\<enter B2 here\> _____

_____, and

\<enter B3 here\> _____

_____.

- But it's important to me to share this thing with you because I hope that sharing it will...

\<enter C1 here\> _____

_____, and

\<enter C2 here\> _____

_____, and

\<enter C3 here\> _____

_____.

- The thing that I want to share with you is…

\<enter A1 here\> _____

_____

_____

_____.

● What do you think?

Appendix C – Love Languages Test

Do this one yourself: Read both statements and circle the one that is strongest for you.

1. A. I love receiving little love notes from you.
   E. I love getting hugs from you.

2. B. I love spending alone time with you.
   D. I love it when you help me with things.

3. C. I love receiving gifts from you.
   B. I love going on walks together.

4. D. I love it when you do things to help me.
   E. I love it when you cuddle me.

5. E. I love it when we snuggle.
   C. I love it when you give me surprise gifts.

6. B. I love going on adventures with you.
   E. I love it when we hold hands.

7. A. I love it when you acknowledge my efforts.
   C. I love it when you give me presents.

8. E. I love it when we sit close enough to touch.
   A. I love it when you tell me you're attracted to me.

9. B. I love spending time alone together.
   C. I love getting little gifts occasionally.

10. D. I love it when you help me with things.
    A. I love it when you tell me you love me.

11. B. I love doing things together with you.
    A. I love when you tell me how you feel.

12. E. I feel awesome when we cuddle.
    D. Your actions are stronger than your words.

13. A. I love your praise.
    C. I love receiving frequent small gifts.

14. E. I feel more love when we touch a lot.
    B. I feel more love when we do things together.

15. A. I love when you praise my achievements.
    D. I feel your love when you do things for me.

16. E. I love it when you touch me a lot through the day.
    B. I love it when you listen attentively to me.

17. C. I love when you surprise me with presents.
    D. I love it when you help me with our to-do list.

18. A. I love it when you compliment me.
    B. I love it when you try to understand me.

19. E. I feel safe when we are touching.
    D. I love it when you do things for me.

20. D. I value everything you do to love me.
    C. I love it when you make me presents.

21. B. I love having your undivided attention.
    D. I love how I feel when you do things for me.

22. C. I love it when you give me presents.
    A. I love it when you tell me how you love me.

23. D. I love it when you help with the chores.
    C. I love it when you give me thoughtful things.

24. C. I love it when you give me things on special days.
    A. I love it when you listen to me patiently.

25. B. I love going on adventures with you
    D. I love it when you help with tasks.

26. E. I love it when you kiss me.
    C. I love it when you surprise me with presents.

27. A. I love hearing that you appreciate me.
    B. I love it when you focus on me.

28. C. I love how your gifts make me feel.
    E. I feel loved when you kiss me.

29. A. I love when you tell me how you love me.
    D. I love it when you do something I ask.

30. E. I love having hugs every day.
    A. I love hearing you love me every day.

Add Total Number of Answers Here:

A. ____ Words of Affirmation

B. ____ Quality Time

C. ____Receiving Gifts

D. ____ Acts of Service

E. ____Physical Touch

The language with the highest number is your primary love language.

Have your partner do this one: Read each pair of statements and circle the one that is the stronger of the two.

1. A. I love receiving little love notes from you.
E. I love getting hugs from you.

2. B. I love spending alone time with you.
D. I love it when you help me with things.

3. C. I love receiving gifts from you.
B. I love going on walks together.

4. D. I love it when you do things to help me.
E. I love it when you cuddle me.

5. E. I love it when we snuggle.
C. I love it when you give me surprise gifts.

6. B. I love going on adventures with you.
E. I love it when we hold hands.

7. A. I love it when you acknowledge my efforts.
C. I love it when you give me presents.

8. E. I love it when we sit close enough to touch.
A. I love it when you tell me you're attracted to me.

9. B. I love spending time alone together.
C. I love getting little gifts occasionally.

10. D. I love it when you help me with things.
A. I love it when you tell me you love me.

11. B. I love doing things together with you.
A. I love when you tell me how you feel.

12. E. I feel awesome when we cuddle.
D. Your actions are stronger than your words.

13. A. I love your praise.
C. I love receiving frequent small gifts.

14. E. I feel more love when we touch a lot.
B. I feel more love when we do things together.

15. A. I love when you praise my achievements.
D. I feel your love when you do things for me.

16. E. I love it when you touch me a lot through the day.
B. I love it when you listen attentively to me.

17. C. I love when you surprise me with presents.
D. I love it when you help me with our to-do list.

18. A. I love it when you compliment me.
B. I love it when you try to understand me.

19. E. I feel safe when we are touching.
D. I love it when you do things for me.

20. D. I value everything you do to love me.
C. I love it when you make me presents.

21. B. I love having your undivided attention.
D. I love how I feel when you do things for me.

22. C. I love it when you give me presents.
A. I love it when you tell me how you love me.

23. D. I love it when you help with the chores.
C. I love it when you give me thoughtful things.

24. C. I love it when you give me things on special days.
A. I love it when you listen to me patiently.

25. B. I love going on adventures with you
D. I love it when you help with tasks.

26. E. I love it when you kiss me.
C. I love it when you surprise me with presents.

27. A. I love hearing that you appreciate me.
B. I love it when you focus on me.

28. C. I love how your gifts make me feel.
E. I feel loved when you kiss me.

29. A. I love when you tell me how you love me.
D. I love it when you do something I ask.

30. E. I love having hugs every day.
A. I love hearing you love me every day.

Add Total Number of Answers Here:

A. _____ Words of Affirmation

B. _____ Quality Time

C. _____Receiving Gifts

D. _____ Acts of Service

E. _____Physical Touch

The language with the highest number is your primary love language.

Appendix D – Pleasure Map Exercise

The pleasure map exercise is very useful to help you learn how your partner likes to receive pleasure. You can use it in many different ways--for example, to learn how your partner likes to receive oral sex or to learn how she likes to receive a hand job. Used once, it helps you learn any single way that she likes to be pleasured. But by copying and printing out the page multiple times, you can use it to learn lots of different ways that she likes to be pleasured. In cases when she doesn't know how to diagram how she likes to be pleasured, it can also be used to help her figure out what she likes!

One of the great things about this exercise is that it helps de-trigger the conversation about what she likes. In other words, it helps to make the conversation about what she likes normal, i.e. to "normalize it." When you can make it easy to talk about her pleasure map, an entire world of possibilities opens up to you both.

Often people are "locked up" and can't discuss openly what they like and dislike, and what they refuse to do and what they'd like to do. By using this exercise in a caring, supportive non-pressuring way, you can open the door to discussing sexual preferences, boundaries, pleasure patterns and sequences that really *work* for your partner. With that valuable information you are then empowered to love and please your partner in the ways that she likes best.

It's a way to gain the information on how to really

"win" with her, and when you demonstrate your interest in learning about her you actively show her that you care. Nothing is more conducive to deepening intimacy and sexual pleasure with a woman than demonstrating to her how much you care for her. That said, these worksheets are intended to offer a general idea of a starting point on her pleasure road map. They should be useful navigational assistance but should not be considered a hard and fast script that you must follow.

Here are a few examples of ways that this worksheet can be used to illustrate pleasure patterns that a woman may find deeply satisfying. These are examples of common patterns that many women like. They are intended to give you an idea of how to use this worksheet as well as better understand some basic pleasure patterns.

Example 1: Shows the steps for one common sequence:

1. Caress and tease the inner thighs and outer labia.

2. Lick and tease the clitoral hood with the tongue.

3. Lick, kiss and suck on the outer labia.

4. Flick the clitoral head left and right directly with the tongue.

5. Insert a finger into the vagina and massage the G-spot while continuing with #4.

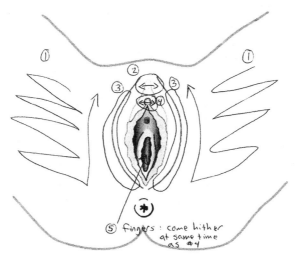

Example 1

Example 2: Shows a way one woman likes to be pleasured after she's already extremely aroused and wet and wants to be vigorously directly stimulated.

- Tongue stimulating clit while two or three fingers move up and down (toward belly button and toward tailbone) inside her vagina.

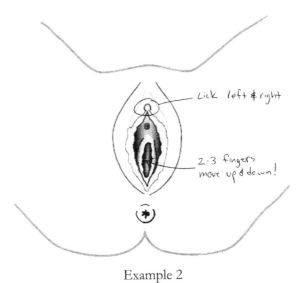

Example 2

Example 3: Shows how one woman likes to receive oral sex with a tongue moving in circular and spiral motions around her entire vulva, clitoris and vaginal opening repeatedly.

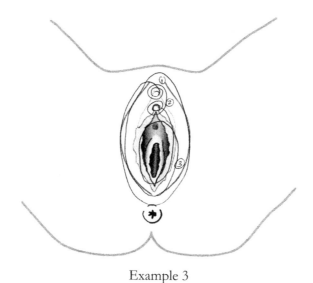

Example 3

Example 4: Shows a way that helps one woman to achieve orgasm with two hands.

- Left hand's first two fingers moving in small circles on her clitoris while…

- Right hand's fingers are inside her vagina moving up and down (toward belly button and toward tailbone).

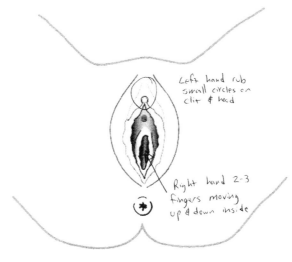

Example 4

Pleasure Map Worksheet (Feel free to copy!):

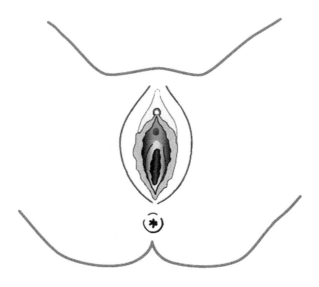

Appendix E –
What If She Doesn't Know
What She Likes?

Throughout this book I repeat the mantras "ask her" and "check in with her" and "let her be your guide." Those are guiding principles that you should engrain in your consciousness and make a habit. But sometimes she may respond and say, "I don't know."

What do you do then?

Some women have more sexual and erotic experience than others. Some women are further along their road of sexual/erotic self-development and mastery. Some women know themselves well: what they like and don't like, how they like to be touched, what makes them orgasm, etc.… Some women have never had anyone in their lives be nice enough to ask them what they like, and other women have little or zero sexual experience at all, so they don't even know what they like or don't like.

So, what do you do?

The answer is: be her ally.

For example, if you are asking her how she likes to receive oral sex, and she says, "I don't know," then you have an amazing opportunity before you. If you become her ally and support, then you may be able to have great fun together! You can ask her if she'd like to explore and try a few different techniques with you because you'd like to learn what pleases her best. You can ask her to do something simple by saying, "I like that a lot," when you find something that she really likes and say, "I don't like that too much," when you do something that doesn't feel that great to her. If you model it for her and tell her that you'd like it if she did that for you, then she may be able to give herself permission to do it.

Another thing that you can do is tell her that you'd like to support her to learn what she likes in a playful way, and that you think that the best way for her to learn what she likes is to masturbate. Ask her if she'd be open to masturbating either alone or with you there so that she can learn how she likes to be touched and where she likes to be touched. If you are there then you get to watch and learn, but she might be too self-conscious to really let go and relax. So, invite her to masturbate alone more and tell you what she learns.

You can even get her a vibrator to help! The Hitachi Magic Wand is a tried and true favorite among women everywhere, and it has helped thousands of women find their orgasms and favorite pleasure pathways.

Lastly, if she says, "I don't know," you can always respond by simply saying, "OK, can we explore this together and see if we can find out what is the most pleasurable to you? Just let me know if I do anything that's really amazing or anything that you'd like me to stop or change!" Aim to keep the channels of communication open and flowing so that you can be in a dialog about what works, what doesn't and what could be improved.

References

Chapter 3 is inspired by the Cuddle Party model of consent and Monique Darling's book, *Beyond Cuddle Party*.

Chapters 4 and 25 are based on by the "Difficult Conversation Formula" by Reid Mihalko.

Chapter 8 is based on *The Five Love Languages* by Dr. Gary Chapman, and the quiz in Appendix D is based on his *Five Love Languages Test*.

Chapter 9 is inspired by *Women's Anatomy of Arousal* by Sheri Winston, CNM.

The described effects of overall fitness (cardiovascular health) on male sexual function are based on "Sexual dysfunction and cardiovascular diseases: a systematic review of prevalence" by Nascimento ER, Maia AC, Pereira V, Soares-Filho G, Nardi AE & Silva AC. Available at the US National Library of Medicine, PMCID: PMC3812559.

The study referenced in Chapter 17, titled "Does Semen Have Antidepressant Properties?" was authored by G. Jr. Gallup in 2002. It can be found in the *Archives of sexual behavior*.

The research on nipple stimulation brain activity in Chapter 18, titled "Women's clitoris, vagina, and cervix mapped on the sensory cortex: fMRI evidence." was authored by Dr. Barry Komisaruk at Rutgers University and published in the *Journal of Sexual Medicine* in 2011.

Chapter 22, 23 and 24 are based on the Removing All Negativity exercise, Reromanticizing exercise, and Imago Dialog, respectively, which were developed by Dr. Harville Hendrix and published in his book, *Getting the Love You Want*.

About the Author

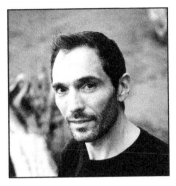

Kristopher Lovestone is a relationship skills instructor, sex educator and men's empowerment facilitator. Originally from St. Louis, Missouri, he now lives in Costa Rica with his family.

He enjoys sailing, para-gliding, strong Costa Rican coffee and geeking out on relationship success strategies.

He teaches and speaks on topics ranging from authenticity tools, boundaries and consent, modern accurate sex education, relationship design, the anatomy of arousal and self-empowerment through finding your inner truth.

His amazingly successful long-term relationship with his wife/best friend is a testament to the value and merit of the tools he teaches--as he lives by example and provides a truly inspiring real-world model of success for his students to follow in their own relationships.

His classes, workshops, online courses, retreats, men's circles and online community, the *Conscious Cock Brotherhood*, help men to rise into the healthy masculine in an empowered and deeply fulfilling way with the essential support of other men.

Find him online at: **www.consciouscock.com**

Made in the USA
Middletown, DE
03 January 2021

30740037R00136